BATS IN MY BELFRY

Dr Bernard Preston

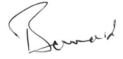

Pen Press Publishers Ltd

First published in Great Britain by
Pen Press Publishers Ltd
The Old School Road
39 Chesham Road
Brighton BN2 1NB

ISBN10: 1-905621-37-X
(ISBN13: 978-1-905621-37-8)

Cover design by Barry Maitland Stuart

For more information about the author go to;
www.bernardpreston.com

Acknowledgements

Many persons have made invaluable contributions to this book, too many to mention. I would like them all to know I have not forgotten. First and foremost, to Jean Jacobi and $ue Halsey, who worked so hard at the manuscript, and trying to understand me, my sincere thanks. Without them, this book would never have found approval from a publisher. My sincere appreciation to the staff at Pen Press Publishers, London with special thanks to Lynn Ashman, Grace Rafael and Linda Harris for their support of a new author.

For the generous donation of their time I would like to acknowledge Dr James Winterstein, President of the National University of Health, and several of his faculty, as well as Dr Barry Lewis, President of the British Chiropractic Association, and thank them for their important contributions.

To two artists extraordinaire, Lorraine Harrison and Barry Maitland-Stuart I would like to say that I am convinced that it is the painstaking work of the artists that finishes a book and gives it a good feel. Thank you.

To Dr Jane

*No man could ask for a finer daughter,
and your decision to follow in my footsteps, and your
grandparents', makes me a very proud man.*

Foreword

I considered it a privilege to have had the opportunity to read the book titled Frog in my Throat by Bernard Preston. It was intriguing and witty and funny and I very much enjoyed it. Now we have the second book by the same author and it is equally insightful and, at the same time, delightful.

Writing about one's professional life might be thought to be easy, but in the doctor/patient relationship, the lines of appropriateness are not always clear, so even without actual names, the care given to this kind of story must be thoughtful and precise.

With this background I once again opened expectantly the pages of Dr Preston's life as a Chiropractic doctor in his relationships and experiences with his patients, his practice, his friends and his family. I was not let down. Again, I was delighted with his stories and often, I found myself thinking of this or that patient whom I had seen during my active practice years.

The practice of a physician, whether Chiropractic or allopathic or other is at once extremely demanding and at the same time so very rewarding. The circumstances with which patients present for care, the situations in which they are entangled and the intrigue of the diagnostic effort, not to mention the therapeutic one are all part of this wonderful little book called Bats in my Belfry.

Whether the reader is a professional health care worker, a Chiropractic student or patient, or indeed anyone from any walk of life, this book will come alive as the pages are turned and the stories become real, from the simple to the funny to the sad, this is a book about people and their true-life circumstances. It is also a book about the care, wisdom, ability and concern of a dedicated doctor of Chiropractic. Perhaps I loved this book because I too am a Chiropractic physician but all who pick it up will relate, will laugh, cry and keep on reading right to the end.

James F. Winterstein, D.C., D.A.C.B.R.
President
National University of Health Sciences

Author's Preface

Such is our human nature, our desire to be loved and approved of, that there is a temptation for a writer to detail only that which may find approval in the eyes of his readers. However, there is another side to us all; one which is rather darker and sometimes shocking, but also more honest and thus I hope worthier of reading.

Do chiropractors make mistakes? Are they open to temptation? Do they have weaknesses? Could they be dreaming about the golf course during a consultation? I won't here bore you in this preface with the character of Bernard Preston, D.C.; that I hope will be self-explanatory in the pages that lie ahead, as you are invited into the intimacy of his consulting room and his private life.

This book will also expose you to something of the Chiropractic universe that is only now in the twenty-first century beginning to unfold, with some 100,000 doctors of Chiropractic worldwide. Owing to some of the uncritical enthusiasm of early chiropractors, and the uninformed denial of the validity of manipulation by medicine, Chiropractic has developed as an apart profession. Today, however, Chiropractic has forged an accepted place in the healthcare market place, a position validated by research and acknowledged by a rapidly expanding part of medicine, including the World Health Organisation.

But mostly, this is a light-hearted fun book that I hope you will enjoy and find inspiring. It dwells on the quirky nature of our human condition, that which is odd, peculiar and sometimes painful. It attempts to show how the ordinary person can be healthier and happier without becoming a radical health-nut or religious fanatic.

Books are rather like money: to generate interest and grow in value they must circulate. I would rather one person bought my books and lent them to twenty friends, than two people bought them and left them gathering dust on a bookshelf. That is a double waste: that space should be reserved only for those treasures that we know we will return to again and again. Feel free to pass *Bats in my Belfry* on to as many friends and family as you like. And, of course, to your medical doctor too!

Dr Bernard Preston, D.C. (Doctor of Chiropractic)

Chapter One

THE DARK NIGHT OF
BERNARD PRESTON'S SOUL

*There will come a time when
you believe everything is finished.
That will be the beginning.*

Louis L'Amour

There was only one fly in all the ointment being massaged into my troubled soul: our cabin neighbours (with whom I had become acquainted whilst fishing on the lake) invited Helen and me over to share a couple of barbecued trout and a glass of wine for lunch. He was going on about the chase and how the trout had ducked into the weeds, routinely tearing up old newspapers for the fire, when he came across the unmistakable picture of his guest. I had read the headline hundreds of times and, even crinkled and upside down, I recognized it immediately: CHIROPRACTOR ACCUSED OF INDECENTLY ASSAULTING SCHOOLGIRL BEAUTY. With a cry, I fled.

It was the Prestons' annual pilgrimage to Lake Pastel, this time not just for a weekend but a whole ten days for refreshment of spirit and restoration of soul. However, that first night found me wide-eyed at two in the morning, watching a bat winging its way amongst the creosoted rafters of the thatched cottage. I idly watched as the furry creature swooped this way and that, desperately trying to find its way out, unable to see the sliding door that I had opened, beckoning freedom.

It was much like being at Wimbledon: Hewitt serves, Federer returns crosscourt, Hewitt rushes to the net but his volley is weak and Federer coolly hits a winner down the line. Back and forth my head turned until I began to wonder if I would get a stiff neck. But my neck seemed to relish the exercise and my mind was mesmerised, relieved, by the tiny mammal flitting amongst the rafters of the cottage that was to become my chapel, its soaring roof, the belfry. The bat? Yes, that bat, became my healer. Or, at least, a start. All great journeys, especially that which seeks to go within, have a first step, humble though it may be.

Habit had trapped the furry creature: instinctively it swooped upwards every time it approached the wall or even the open door, saving its head, but also not finding the great outdoors that it was so earnestly seeking. I wondered how many nights it had been haphazardly flitting about, trapped, and how long it could survive without food and water. What had induced this poor blind creature, free to twist and turn in the night sky darting about after its dinner, to fly into this bat-trap? Had he sold his soul for a mere mosquito? *A mess of pottage*?* Just what had drawn him in? It was not long before I made the connection to my own reality; what had sucked me into my man-trap, my self-made folly, my own blindness?

For three wakeful nights that bat and I shared each other's company. I watched him and exercised my neck and he, I suppose, sensed me apprehensively with his radar. Finally, during my third sleepless night, just as the first tinges of salmon pink fingered the mountains, and even mighty Sirius began to fade, I realized his swoops were beginning to weaken. No longer could he rise upwards in his instinctive manner as he approached the wall and, just as I was wondering whether the fishing net might save his life, he shot

---

* Biblical metaphor: Esau sold his birthright to his brother Isaac for a pot of beans.

out the still-open door to life. *L'chaim.*[*] To life. Instinct had trapped him but finally, in his weakness, he found life and freedom.

Those wretched nights I had found myself waking, soon after I had fallen asleep, with only that bat for company. Helen, perhaps surprisingly, was in a deep and seemingly untroubled sleep. For ten long years, ignoring her pleas, I had taken little more than a few days of leave, sporadically snatched here and there, and I was desperately exhausted. Bitter, restless nights of tossing and turning followed. I was estranged from my wife and my God was hidden on the other side of a leaded heaven. I had become a stranger to those who loved me, lost in a dark maze of depression and tormented by the eyes of the beautiful young woman who had mesmerised me. There appeared to be no escape. The demand to appear before the disciplinary Chiropractic Board[†] to explain my conduct had been the final straw, crushing my already bruised and exhausted spirit. Reality was dealing with me. Summonsing all my willpower I applied for three teaching posts at local high schools, confident that I could find employment as a science teacher and fled to Lake Pastel Mountain Resort – only to find a bat, and a new beginning.

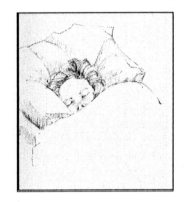

Instinct. Aim higher. Work harder. You're not pushing yourself enough, Bernie. You must earn more. Time to take up that post as chairman of the local Chiropractic branch.

---

[*] Used in Jewish toasts, 'l' meaning 'to' and 'chaim' meaning 'life'.
[†] Reference: *Frog in my Throat.*

3

Foot flat. Pedal on the right. What's the matter, Bernie? Are you okay?

'No, I'm not okay. And I'm no longer a chiropractor. I've sacked myself. I'm going back to teaching 'cause the Chiropractic shoe is pinching my foot. Okay?'

The episode of the beautiful young model, not even out of school, had collapsed my world. She had targeted me, mesmerising me with her beautiful eyes and I had been helplessly caught in her web, or so it seemed in my wretched state of mind. In actual fact my conduct had been above reproach, although my thoughts were certainly more suspect.

The Board had ultimately found me not guilty but, in my depressed state, I was doomed: hooked, reeled in and netted by the young woman, still technically only a child. Then I had been gutted and hung out to dry like a trophy by the press. Now it felt as though my head was about to be crudely guillotined with a heavy fishing knife. Dark, depressed images flooded my mind as rational thought fled. I was a complete failure, to myself, my family and my profession. The black dog was stalking me. *Anne of a Thousand Days*[*] would be my companion. Night after sleepless night I despaired.

What had I done wrong? Yes, I had been attracted to her. Who wouldn't be? I had to admit that; it was true, I had been tempted. But equally true was that, in the end, I had neither done, nor said, anything untoward but I was not in a position to grasp that yet. I was damned. And then the God, whom I could neither see nor find, sent a very tiny bat, weighing less than a few ounces into my life; a starving bat, that flitted back and forwards, night after night, hungry and thirsty whilst trapped in my cottage but never giving up.

He had sold his freedom, in exchange for a mere mosquito. And I? What had I to show for my success?

---

[*] Anne Boleyn, Henry VIII's second wife, who lost her head.

Finally, utterly exhausted, my bat was unable to swoop upwards any longer and had, almost accidentally, found his way out through the open door to freedom.

Freedom and life. Life and freedom. A tiny ray of light shot into the cell of my depression. *It was for freedom that I set you free...*[*] The words, memorised so long ago, came bursting into my mind and, for the first time, I began to realize that I had imprisoned myself, and driven myself almost to madness in my own consulting rooms.

Circumstances had now forced me, close to a complete breakdown, to find a locum and take an extended break; forced me to consider the life of a humble bat flying around the belfry, high up in the 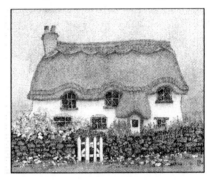 cottage that was to become the chapel where my healing began. Quiet tears of joy began coursing down my cheeks and, when Helen called sleepily through the open bedroom door, I fell into her arms and a deep and dreamless sleep.

The afternoon sun was pouring into the bedroom when I woke to the aroma of fresh coffee, hissing and spitting in the kitchen. Ah, the smell of freshly brewed coffee, much better than the taste really, and not too good for my stressed adrenal glands but just what I needed. A new peace settled over me as I lay in the warm sunshine, the winter rays angled onto our bed, reflecting on the lesson of the bat. He hadn't given up as I had been about to do, yet it was only when he was utterly at the end of his tether that he found the open door. I had some

---

[*] Galations 5:1.

thinking to do. *Was I the owner of my practice, or did my practice...? Who's the boss?*

Thank God for a helpmate who stuck by her man through thick and thin. For better or for worse. Many a woman in her circumstances would have left her husband years ago for greener pastures. Over the second cup I shared the vision of the bat with Helen. It was she, seeing my state of mind, who had forced me to take a month's leave, starting with ten days in the beautiful cottage at Lake Pastel, the original farmhouse built by a Devonshire immigrant. She was very angry at my decision to go back to teaching: 'Do you think we wasted all that time and energy going to Chicago for nothing? Surely you remember that those who can, do, and those who can't...' A teacher herself, she couldn't bring herself to finish the nasty quote but, being more a person of faith than I, Helen didn't stand in the way of my choice. She believed firmly in a God who could open doors that none could shut – and who would shut doors, no matter how badly science teachers were needed. All three schools, as it happened, turned down my applications.

'Ever heard of Robert the Bruce?' she asked me over our cups of coffee. We were sitting on the warm veranda enjoying the view over the lake with the mountains in the background. Helen was Scots, her family coming from Dundee-on-Tay.

'Mm, some Scotsman?'

'Yes, he was king in Edinburgh when King John of England was determined to conquer Scotland. The Scots were defeated in a great battle with the English and the Bruce and his men were routed. He had to hide from the English in a cave.'

'Is this a history lesson, or what?' I was beginning to relax, and asked the question without malice.

'Yes, you and the Bruce have something in common.'

'I thought you said he was pure royalty. I'm only a commoner,' I replied with a laugh. 'What can we possibly have in common?'

'Didn't you know that puns are the lowest form of wit?' she shot back with a smile, tossing a serviette at me. 'The Bruce was skulking in his cave when he saw a spider trying to spin a web across the mouth of the cave. All day the spider swung back and forth, failing time after time, until finally in the early evening the wind changed a point or two, and propelled the persistent creature, dangling from her thread, the extra few centimetres across the cave. By morning the mouth of the cave was covered by her web.'

'Of bats and spiders,' I said, offering my repartee with a laugh. 'Not just of mice and men?'

Helen ignored my comeback: 'The Bruce was so inspired that he rallied his men and they went on to defeat the English. I'll leave you to work out the moral of the story!'

We went for a quiet walk around the lake, watching several fishermen trying their luck, soaking in the late afternoon sunshine, and listening to the frogs beginning their courting. The trout were coming on the rise, but I was in no mood to cast a fly. It was nearly a week before my favourite sport began to appeal.

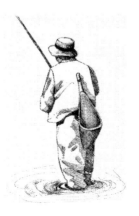

With each step I could feel the tension in my shoulders beginning to relax and Helen's arm around my waist reassured my stressed spirit. She had also been hurt by the saga of the model, and the gentle squeeze of her arm meant a great deal to me.

Later, we sat on the veranda of the clubhouse sipping our nondescript dry sherries as the sun sank over the Rhino mountain peak, the distinctive horn shape silhouetted against the evening sky. The Drakensberg chain of mountains reaches a modest eleven thousand feet and its snowy cap began to chill the evening air. Suddenly, there was a sound of flapping wings behind my head, the shriek of an angry bird, and a wing brushed my ear. I raised my arm protectively but the mother did me no harm. I looked up at the nest of Red-wing Starlings just above our heads; young chicks were poking out their heads, shrilly calling for more worms. It brought back memories.

'Did I ever tell you about Harry Singh who lost an eye?' I asked Helen. She was silently enjoying the far horizons.

'No, I don't think so. An Indian I presume. How did it happen?' she said, turning to me.

'There was a wind-storm in Swartberg late one afternoon and an Indian Mynah chick was blown out of its nest. Harry went to rescue the tiny bird and the enraged mother flew down and pecked out his eye.'

'That's dreadful, but how did he end up in your clinic?'

'That was a couple of years later. He stepped on a leaf of lettuce in his supermarket and fell on his buttocks and slipped a disc.'

'So who is going to fix Mr Singh's back the next time he does himself a mischief after you have gone back to teaching?' Helen asked, after a few moments of thought. I remained silent, still unaware that three rejections of my applications were in the post, thinking about the irony of an Indian man trying to save the exotic chick, and having his eye pecked out by an irate mother. Questions of race, its

8

injustices and ironies, occupy the thoughts of all South Africans. On the racial roller-coaster, I pondered as I watched Sacred Ibis and Hadedas* sharing the wide expanse of lawn stretching down to the lake and a Grey Heron and a Kingfisher spearing fingerlings and tadpoles peacefully within a few metres of each other. A flock of fifty Guineafowl, only twenty metres away, was scratching and hunting for crickets. True, there was a Shrike and a Bulbul squabbling over the same worm, but they didn't kill each other! Why couldn't we humans live and let live? Although not any sort of ornithologist, even I was fully aware that Starlings and Indian Mynas were first cousins. I had been lucky to get away with just a warning from the angry mother. *Chicks can be dangerous*, I thought.

It was another four days before I could cast a fly into the lake. I was dimly aware that depression takes the joy out of even favourite activities. I was down, no doubt about it. *Burnout.* Quietly, I pushed out on the flat-bottomed boat, taking my time, unhurried, relishing the moment. The oars squeaked in their locks but I hardly noticed. Opening my box of flies I savoured the choosing of the first fly. Looking at the sky and then the water I carefully selected a Walker Killer and tied it onto my line. The sun had already sunk over the mountains and I sat back, drinking in the peace and the calm. I could think of no other place on earth that I would rather be: the sky, the lake, the birds and the fish. Were there any fish? I took in a deep breath, cherishing the tangible tranquillity. A half moon grew steadily in intensity, the last of the fading sunset still reflected on the glassy waters of the lake, doubly enjoyed. It was pure magic and I bowed my head, giving thanks for the great gift of creation. I had learnt not to worship creation; instead I silently honoured the Creator for his great gift. Why else did He make this

---

* Large noisy Ibis that wakens the world, typical of Southern Africa.

wondrous place, if not for mere mortals to enjoy and be restored? Bats were flitting about the evening sky and I wondered if my friend was amongst them, winging his way above my head. I had opened a door to freedom for him. And he? Well, he had opened another door for me. We needed each other, that bat and I.

My first casts were unproductive. No fish took the fly but, with each throw of the heavy line, I could feel the depression and the exhaustion gradually fading, like the day, into the lake and sky. The moonlight twinkled in the ripples around my line and the occasional sound of a trout rising was ointment to my tormented soul. That first hour no trout troubled my fishing net but I relished the palpable restoration.

A particularly feeble cast dropped the tangled line just a few metres from the boat. Unhooking my line in the near dark allowed the fly to sink deep into the lake. Whilst I was fumbling with the knot, suddenly a savage tug brought me to my feet and, with a shout of exultation, I began to play the fish. He was no great monster but he would feed us tonight and, as I netted him, I knew that, for the time being the black dog had left me.

It was quite dark when I arrived back at the tiny cottage. Helen gave a groan when she saw the fish. She too was tired.

'Let's go over to the clubhouse and see if the kitchen staff won't cook it for us,' I suggested.

'Certainly, Doctor,' the maître d' said. He was a tall and handsome Zulu man. In his black uniform with a tiny silver trout on his chest, he cut a fine figure. Damn! How had he discovered that I was in the healing professions? I valued my privacy and I had come to this remote place to escape the doctoring business.

We sat quietly in a corner enjoying a bottle of Helen's favourite, a Boschendal *le Bouquet*, looking out of the open window over the lake, with the half moon still reflected on the waters. Half moon, half healed? I banished the thought. Only the frogs and a distant owl calling to its mate disturbed the night air, as we waited for our dinner, knowing it would take a while to prepare. Quietly we held hands, rejoicing in the life that was beginning to flow again through my veins, when there was a shout.

'Doctor, doctor, please come!' Reluctantly I looked up. 'A man is choking. He is dying. Please come!' The maître'd pulled urgently at my sleeve.

I looked at Helen and she gave me a tiny nod. I rose quickly, picking up a steak knife, ready to do a tracheotomy. Third tracheal ring rang a bell. As I followed the handsome Zulu to the smoking section, screened off by heavy plate glass doors, my mind quickly settled back into action mode. Fortunately, the steak knife was not needed. (Most fortunately as I had neither done nor even seen a tracheotomy being done, except on video more than twenty years earlier. An anathema to every non-medical first-aid student, the thought of cutting a man's throat terrified me but the experienced paramedic had firmly made his point: *'Be prepared to do it or watch the man die in front of you in little more than two minutes.'*). The man was gagging, clutching his throat, still sitting on his bench, utterly unable to gasp even the smallest breath. His wife was screaming in terror. I quickly checked his vital signs, noting his already blue, oxygen-starved lips, glad that I did an annual refresher course of basic First Aid. There were no sounds of breath so, leaning him forwards, I gave him five hefty thumps on the back. It made not the slightest difference. Calling for help, two strong men quickly came to my aid, supporting the choking man as he passed out. Absurdly, I was distracted momentarily by the enormous thick steak, neatly sitting in the centre of a silver salver with only one large piece sliced out. The piece firmly stuck in his windpipe, I thought, wolfed down by the apparently starving man. I reached around him giving him a violent Heimlich thrust into the solar plexus with my fist, rolling the wrist to increase the sharp jab against the diaphragm. He gave a choking sound as the piece of steak burst from his windpipe and he started to gag, gasping for breath. We laid him on the floor on his side making sure that he didn't choke again, while I cleaned the vomit and the large piece of rump out of his mouth with my finger, the handle of the steak knife firmly wedged between his teeth. I didn't want to lose a finger. Chiropractors need all ten. Teachers, too. Again I checked his vital signs. All were intact. He was breathing normally again and it was not long before he recovered consciousness. Helen and I slipped quietly away, our trout forgotten.

Helen squeezed my arm in the dark as we walked back to our cottage: 'You saved a man's life tonight.'

'Just as well it was tonight, not last night,' I muttered. 'Yesterday I would have just left him to die.'

But the following day I fled the resort in terror, my past inescapable. For years I broke out in a sweat if someone started tearing up newspapers.

Chapter Two

THE INSIDE STORY

I'm still learning.

Michaelangelo, aged 85

I had enormous respect for the old man. One of my colleagues had once whispered in my ear: 'If you can't get a back right, refer them to Dr Coulter before you send them for surgery.' He was right. Chiropractic, perhaps like all of medicine and in fact life itself, is an admixture of science and art, and Dr Coulter was one of those who had perfected the chemistry. Of course at 79 years of age, he had been in practice for over fifty years; my twenty-seven, in comparison, had a very miserly look about them. Most things, but not all, are relative. Nevertheless, I had to ask myself the question: Would I be any better a chiropractor after thirty-seven years in practice, and after forty-seven years? What was it that would make me better? More science? More conferences and seminars? More lectures on the philosophy of Chiropractic?

When the invitation to dinner with Dr Coulter and his wife arrived I was determined not to miss the evening. Helen and I dressed carefully. She looks stunning in long dresses with bright, large floral patterns: the deep pink Rhododendrons, laced with silver thread on a purple background and my mother's pearls did her proud. With her long legs she looked lovely. Every man is proud when he can hum, as I did that evening: *Pretty woman, walking beside me...* Gone were the short, black party dresses that the maths student once wore. The occasion was described as 'smart casual' and for once I actually thought about what I was going to wear. Glider pilots for some reason are completely disdainful of such things. *Wereld se goed;*[*] we are proudly of another world which has its own sartorial ideas. Eventually I settled for grey pants, smartly ironed with all the creases neatly showing down the front, a long-sleeved white shirt and a dark navy-blue double-breasted jacket and tie.

I had often mused over home practices. They have their demerits... but the thought of not having to drive to work... and owning only one car and my *dream machine*[*] would be more than adequate for us. Only one telephone and one electricity bill. I sighed, starting to add up the reasons why I should be moving my practice to High Whytten. One rates account. Even if only half my patients were prepared to drive up the hill, I would still be better off financially, and I could do carpentry two afternoons a week! I was determined to see what made Dr Coulter's home practice tick.

We saw the sign emblazoned at the door: CONSULTATION BY APPOINTMENT ONLY. Dr Coulter himself answered the doorbell: 'Welcome. Welcome my dear, you look splendid,' he said to Helen in the gracious way of a generation now nearly gone. A few relics remain to remind the barbarians that there is another way of living.

I noticed the half drunk glass of beer on the table next to the door. Helen noticed it too. One of our rules was: Never start drinking before the guests arrive and for me the first drink had to be soft. Quite often the first two actually, because they don't even touch sides after a long day in the air. Helen gave me a meaningful glance and raised an eyebrow. We had been over this ground before, many times: Bernard Preston, on occasion, drank too much. That's the problem of having a carboy of mead bubbling in one corner

---

[*] Worldly goods (Afrikaans).

[*] Bernard Preston's large BMW motorcycle. See *Frog in my Throat*.

14

of the kitchen and a cask of beer giving off aromatic gurgles in another.

Our host offered us drinks, but I noticed that he had only a glass of sparkling water with a squeeze of fresh lemon and a few mint leaves. Helen and I circulated in the small crowd of chiropractors and their spouses, all of whom I knew well. It was interesting to note that nearly half of the chiropractors were women. Some patients foolishly don't want a woman chiropractor. *How can they have the strength to do what you do?* During my earliest days in practice I had noticed how my senior colleague could adjust almost any back that I could. Perhaps once a month she might send me a huge bear of a man who was too big for her but it was no more often than that. In fact, I eventually realized that women very often make better chiropractors than men, because they are obliged to use skill and timing rather than brute force and ignorance. Every South African can think of diminutive people like Gary Player or the Rose of Soweto[*] who have become great sportsmen. They could hit a golf ball or sting like a bee just as sweetly as any of the giants and were often a lot faster around the field or the ring. Could unskilled, overly forceful or thoughtlessly done Chiropractic adjustments injure a spine? What a foolish question.

I stayed close to the old man as I watched him being attentive to his guests. I thought to myself: *I bet he treats his patients with the same courtesy.* Mrs Coulter was bringing in traditional delights, and I noticed another younger woman, her daughter-in-law as it happened, was helping. They had been hard at work since early morning whilst I was out enjoying a halcyon day, soaring the hot summer skies. Despite the fact we were colleagues, he thirty years older than I, I had continued to call him Doc. Everybody did, even his wife. Dr Coulter poured the ladies each a glass of wine, a white and a red from the fairest Cape, and I saw him pour

---

[*] Famous diminutive South African sportsmen.

15

what was no doubt his first whisky. A half shot with plenty of ice. I matched him with my first beer. My tongue was hanging out.

John, a colleague from the next village, button-holed me. 'You know, Bernie, Jack Stott is taking the most appalling x-rays. I asked him to send me the file of a patient who had moved to Swartberg. If I had had to mail out those films to a colleague, I would have made up some lie and contrived to lose them. If the medics saw them they would tear strips off us.' I had had words with Jack Stott when he had first moved to Shafton, and nicknamed him Jack Sprat; his wife Noleen was, however, a darling. She is Australian and, despite our disastrous introduction, she and Helen had become firm friends. I heard Helen's gay high-pitched laugh and, glancing over saw them enjoying a private joke.*

'To be quite honest, John, I am considering selling my old machine for just that reason. Now that the Rad labs will take x-rays for us, and the medical insurance will then pay for them, I suspect the taking of x-rays by chiropractors will become a dying procedure. By the time I've paid for all the expenses, I reckon my machine costs me money.'

John nodded. 'Yes, that may be true.'

'On the other hand,' I said, 'chiropractors have been at the forefront of developing new screens and filters. It's something the profession should discuss. I wonder which will be the first college to take the dramatic step of no longer teaching radiography.'

'Oh, I doubt if it'll come to that,' said John, hastily. 'I really value how quickly I can get a set of x-rays. I would never part with my machine.'

I thought of how I could get a set of films back, with a Radiologist's report, in a couple of hours. I would gladly ditch my machine. I could then treat another couple of patients in the time it took to take and develop those films,

---

* Reference: *Frog in my Throat.*

instead of having to work such long hours. Adjusting spines was what excited me, not taking x-rays. I held my tongue, keeping my opinions to myself for a change.

'Mind you,' I went on, 'I wonder if it's not like computers. Just as they have evolved, even dropping the floppy drives, and I suspect the CD drive in the not too distant future, I have a suspicion that Chiropractic education will evolve, and leave Radiography behind.

John nodded but I could see he wasn't thinking about computers. 'Are you saying that we may soon have a Chiropractic college that will stop teaching x-ray? What about reading x-rays.' My colleague looked at me incredulously.

'Stopping radiography, not radiology. We must continue to excel at reading x-rays.'

'Hmff! Quite a thought. What about the State Boards? You could never pass them without being able to take x-rays.'

'Well, that's obviously a problem but as the number of chiropractors who actually take x-rays gradually drops, I suspect the time will come. Just watch. As for your original question, John: Just go to Jack, take him a drink or something, and in a very friendly manner, tell him what you just told me. We all take bad x-rays sometimes, the radiologists do too. I have had to send patients back for repeats occasionally. When I graduated I still remember old Doc Hough saying: 'Ask yourself this question with every set of x-rays: *If I had to take these to court, could I hold my head up high?*'

We ran out of conversation and, as he made a determined move towards Jack Sprat, I silently wished him good luck, and headed over to the bar. I had seen Doc Coulter pouring his second half shot. I could use another beer, I thought.

'Now that we are all here, can I drink a toast to the chiropractors of...?' There was a loud knock on the front door. Dr Coulter rose and I could see he was visibly irritated. Putting his whisky down, he walked to the door and I watched him pick up the half glass of beer. We couldn't see who was there but we could hear the loud voice. 'Doc, I have a terrible pain in my back. It's been agony for three days and I just can't face another sleepless night.'

'Ah sir, normally I would be very happy to oblige, but I'm afraid once I've had a few drinks I never treat patients. If you've had the pain for three days, then I'm sure it will keep until morning. Would you mind phoning tomorrow and my secretary will make an appointment for you?'

The man started to argue, but the old gentleman went on to give him a few suggestions about ice packs and, if it really was that bad, he had better get over to the emergency rooms. He then firmly closed the door. He put the half glass of beer down again at the front door, and it finally dawned on me: That glass lived there permanently. When I looked at the glass later with interest, I noticed the fruit flies and a small beetle floating in the amber liquid. Lesson number one for a home practice: Learn to say NO when it's important. Firmly, but kindly, and always give an alternative. Later, I got to thinking about getting the balance right between 'I care' and 'I also have my private life'. It was a juggle and, inevitably one would make a fumble or drop the baton occasionally.

'As I was saying: "A toast to the chiropractors of East Griqualand, your spouses and to our other guests. Make yourselves at home and have a wonderful evening."' He raised his glass: 'To our patients and the profession.' There was a chorus from around the room, and I thought to myself: *What a fine toast. This man really has the balance – our patients and the profession, in that order.* There were a few visiting chiropractors from neighbouring KwaZulu Natal so, all in all, we were about twenty-five people. After the toast, the general hub-hub rose again, but it wasn't long before there were angry voices from the far side of the living room.

18

Everybody hushed and turned towards the corner where John and Jack Stott were having a spat.

'How dare you criticize my x-rays!' Jack's angry words sliced through the convivial atmosphere. 'There's nothing wrong with them at all. A damn cheek.'

'Look Jack, I was just trying to point out in a very friendly manner that those x-rays you sent me were not very good.'

'How dare you say they were not good. That's the last set of x-rays I'll ever send you!'

'Okay, okay. I've said my piece. I had no intention of making a scene. I'm sorry I brought it up here. I should have phoned you at the office.'

'No, you should not. No one has the right to criticize my x-rays, not here, nor over the phone. Just mind your own business.' I could see Nolene making her way over towards her husband, firmly taking his elbow, and removing the drink from his hand.

'I'm sorry, really I'm sorry,' said my friend, backing away. He went over to our host, and I could see him apologizing for making a scene.

Mrs Coulter, wise like her husband, rang the bell even though dinner wasn't quite ready. 'Time for dinner, everybody, please make your way to the dining room.' Their billiard table, when turned upside down, made a giant dining room table. It was beautifully set for the party, with fresh flowers and napkins carefully folded in a fan. I did my bit for King and Country and took the seat next to Jack. For once I was quite sober, and determined to keep the peace. Noleen was sitting on the far side of him, and I had encouraged Helen to sit next to her friend, opposite me. They didn't have much time to see each other and this was the perfect opportunity. Jack was muttering to himself: 'Damn cheek, damn cheek, *damn* cheek.' I could see him starting to look for a drink, scraping his chair but I was much quicker. 'Can I get you a drink, Jack? You like a whisky with dinner, don't you?'

Noleen glared at me, but I gave her a wink. My favourite uncle had been a hotel manager and I had learnt many of the tricks of the trade from him. One of them, he had assured me, is that a man who has had too much to drink has no idea what he is drinking. If he was really drunk, you could give him a glass of tonic on the rocks and he would believe you if you told him that it was a G and T. This was just the right moment to test his ideas.

I went over to the bar and, with my back to Jack, so that he couldn't see what I was doing, I half filled a glass with ice and soda and a tenth of a tot of whiskey. Taking half a glass of red wine for myself, I walked back to the table, put Jack's drink down in front of him and, to distract him, raised my glass: 'To our host and hostess, thank you for a wonderful evening.' My ruse worked. Jack raised his glass, took a healthy swallow and was none the wiser.

'Thank you, Bernie, that was damn noble of you,' Jack said.

The dinner was uneventful. Once he had an Eland steak inside him, a healthy pile of roast potatoes and an spicy spinach roll, filled with fried onion and melted Feta cheese, Jack behaved himself. We actually had an interesting discussion about heel lifts, and I reluctantly ended up promising to remove some bees from their roof. Mrs Coulter was Dutch and we were introduced to a Limburg vlaai, a large tart with a pastry base, cream cheese and honey filling, all covered with a layer of East Griqualand cherries and a thick sweet cherry sauce. Whipped cream was an option for those like me with no discretion.

After dinner I left Jack to the ladies. Guests were circulating again, enjoying coffee and mint chocolates, and I wanted a word with our host. 'Doc Coulter, could I have a moment?'

'Sure, Bernie. What's up?'

'I've been in practice for twenty-seven years now but I still feel I have so much to learn. Do you think I could spend a couple of hours watching you treat patients?'

'That would be a great pleasure. You are just at the stage where I started to get on top of Chiropractic and it started with two ingredients: first, how much you know you still have to learn. That's not easy for someone who has been in practice for as long as you have.'

I nodded. 'Someone once said: "Being *good* is the greatest enemy of becoming *great*." And secondly?'

'Secondly, an enquiring mind, and that I see you have. Give Joan a call in the morning and we'll set something up.'

'Thank you, that would be wonderful. Secondly, I want to apologise for that little fracas earlier. John asked me what to do, and I suggested he do the honourable thing and approach Jack in a friendly way. I thought it would be much better than a formal complaint.'

'Yes, that's fine. Actually, I have also heard rumours about his shocking x-rays. It's your job as chairman of the peer review committee to do something about it, isn't it?'

'Yes, it is, and frankly I have been weak, and avoiding Jack, because I know there will be a confrontation. Our wives are friends but now I have to do something.'

'Yes, do it before he blackens our good name here in East Griqualand.'

Helen and I bade our farewells, and made our way to the car, after making sure that Jack and Noleen were heading in the same direction. There was an awkward moment as Noleen headed for the driver's seat, but I took Jack's arm: 'Do yourself a favour, Jack and do as the good wife suggests. Good night, Stotts.' I tossed Helen my keys and walked to our car. I never looked back but as we were driving off I was glad to see that Noleen was in the driving seat.

A full bladder and a dry mouth woke me early next morning – I always seem to waken in the *wee* small hours after a few drinks. I sat down and drew up a roster of peer review visits to all the chiropractors in the province, writing my own name at the top of the list. I wrote letters to two colleagues inviting them to join me on the peer review committee, and they were numbers two and three to be reviewed. Dr Coulter would be the chair of those first three assessments. Jack Stott was next.

My visits to Dr Coulter were intended to last a month, but went on for six until he very suddenly died. During those six months I learnt much about the old man, his philosophy of life, the way in which he practised, and how a home practice could be a functional reality. Perhaps the most important was the day when he had been bitten by a spider, and had a very painful wrist.

'Bernie, would you mind treating my patients today, seeing that you are visiting?'

'Why of course, Doc.'

It was an uneventful morning until the last patient. She was a small wiry woman and I was quite unable to adjust her pelvis. After several attempts, using eventually too much force, I gave up and she left, protesting, in more pain than when she arrived.

'Sorry about that, Doc. I'm not sure why I couldn't adjust her back.'

'Yes, I've been watching you all morning, Bernie. May I make a suggestion? Come and lie here on the Pelvic Bench.'

He set me up in the usual way but with subtle changes. 'You are putting too much rotation into the spine. If you take your contact here on the elbow, and take out the traction *cephalad** instead of with so much rotation, then I think you will have better results. Remember to keep the patient's leg straight, too.'

---

* Towards the head.

Those six months with Doc Coulter got me thinking. As branch chairman I invited all of our members to spend a morning with a colleague every six months. Jack Sprat and few others refused but it wasn't long before other report-backs started trickling in, making me realize our richest resource was our own members. It was another five years, though, before that home practice in High Whytten became a reality. The call to do a three-year stint overseas undid all my planning.

Chapter Three

MRS BOUCHER'S MANTRAP

Is not marriage an open question,
when it is alleged, from the beginning of the world
that such as are in the institution wish to get out,
and such as are out wish to get in?

Ralph Emerson 1882

In health practice you have to learn many things the hard way. In fact, your patients usually become your teachers and even on occasion your mentor. If you, like me, are a slow learner, then you especially hope they don't sue you while you are 'practising' – on them.

My daughter's music teacher was the one who taught me that if an older woman falls on her back or buttocks and has lower mid-back pain, then I must take an x-ray. *Always.* For the simple reason that they will often have a compression fracture of the spine, in which case manipulation is definitely inadvisable. Rose had slipped in the garden on wet grass one Sunday morning, landing on her buttocks. By the afternoon she was in considerable pain. Not agony but she was sore. Deep breathing was painful, as was moving her arms and when I percussed on the spine later that afternoon she found it a little painful. Again, not agony but enough to say: *well, it could be...* The other distinct possibility was a cracked or subluxated rib.[*] The problem was that the first two diagnoses

---

[*] The ribs have joints at both ends, both of which can be injured and cause pain in the chest or the back.

definitely meant manipulation was the worst form of treatment. However, for a subluxated rib, manipulation was the treatment of choice. Ah, I hear you say: so *what is your diagnosis, doctor?* That's where I have great difficulty with those chiropractors who say: *We don't diagnose. We only adjust the spine.* I made my diagnosis – and got it wrong.

In those early days, I was not unhappy to treat patients with whom I was not reasonably sure of the diagnosis (after all, is one ever totally sure?). Now I am a little older and, I hope, wiser.

Mistake number one: 'We'll give you a gentle treatment, Rose but, if you're not much better in three days, then we must have an x-ray taken. Are you happy with that?'

'Yes, Bernie, of course, if you think so. I'm in your hands. Literally!' she said with a half-hearted wink. She was hurting.

Bernie thought so, but Bernie was wrong. He should have sent her there and then or at least, being Sunday, first thing next morning to the radiologist, without first treating her.

Mistake number two: Even my relatively gentle mobilisation of the joint aggravated the fracture – *of course,* I hear you say. Yes, of course. I made what could have been a serious mistake, but those were the days before my Golden Rules had been firmly established and formalised in my mind:

Take a good history: I knew she had fallen and could have fractured something.

Do a thorough examination: Possible fracture of a rib or vertebra, possible subluxation of rib-head or spinal joint, possible strain of back muscles (unlikely, as isometric testing was relatively painless), or even a sprain of the supporting ligaments. Or several of the above. Trauma often injures more than one tissue.

Use other tests to confirm diagnosis: that's where Rose had to pay the price for Bernie being equivocal. He was trying to save her the substantial cost of an x-ray; they weren't well off. Most of the music world seems to be disgustingly rich, or really quite poor.

Make the diagnosis and the differential diagnoses (other possibilities).

Only then begin *treatment*.

Well, Rose got better, once I applied the appropriate treatment, and she was largely pain-free within four weeks as long as she was sensible. Fortunately she wasn't unduly hurt by an inexperienced chiropractor messing about and I didn't have to refer her out. Fortunately it wasn't a serious compression, but it was enough to make her miserable for a couple of weeks. Fortunately, I wasn't sued, probably because she was my daughter's music teacher.

Mrs Boucher, on the other hand, made me laugh but ultimately also quite angry. At least I didn't miss the diagnosis.

'Doctor, I have pain in my back.'

'When did it start, Mrs Boucher, did you have a fall or something. Did you lift something heavy?'

'Yes, I fell in the night on the way to the loo.' She wouldn't look me in the eye, and I had the distinct sense that there was more to this fall. I had learnt to follow my intuition by that time – it was usually worth the journey.

'Like to tell me about it?'

'I tripped. Plain and simple!' she snapped and her manner said it all: *don't pry,* but I was in the mood for prying and it might, in any case, be important.

'Was it over your slippers?'

'Mind your own business. I tripped and fell on my buttocks. That's all you need to know.' She might have been eighty plus but that didn't mean Mrs Boucher had lost any of her spirit. She was tiny, prim and proper, her long hair tied back in a bun but still she was a feisty woman; so I got on with it.

Flexion of her spine was very painful and, when I percussed with my reflex hammer, she gave a small cry of pain. The most common place for a fracture is where the highly mobile lumbar spine meets the much more stable thoracic spine (stable because of the ribs). Sure enough, it was the last thoracic vertebra that was so painful.

X-rays confirmed a serious compression fracture of the vertebral body. Fractures of that nature mean bleeding and because of the proximity of the kidneys and ureter, I decided to refer her to the orthopaedic surgeon who had bought Jeremy Thomas's practice, a Mr Sinclair. He was in a far better position to manage the fracture, and any possible sequelae,* being in immediate contact with other specialists. Some specialists still like to be called Mister, a cut above the ordinary Doctor. I also used to stand on my high horse but, after being humbled numerous times, was very happy with plain Bernie Preston.

I got a brief letter from him, confirming that he had booked her into St Augustine's hospital for a few days. Following that, she was to use a corset for at least six weeks, and he expected her to be largely pain-free within two to three months. Well and good, I agreed with his plan of action, and forgot about Mrs Boucher and how she tripped on the way to the loo in the night.

It was some eighteen months later that Mrs Boucher again appeared in my appointment book. I remembered her well, it was an unusual name and she was an unusual person. She hadn't aged much but I could see from the way she walked and sat down that she was in a lot of pain.

'Your back is still hurting, I see, Mrs Boucher. Did the pain never go away, or has it come back? Have you taken another fall on the way to the loo?'

She scowled at me. 'The pain was about fifty per cent better after three months but, ever since then, if I do

---

* Any abnormality following or a disease or injury.

anything, even simple things, it gets very sore.' She moved awkwardly in her chair. 'I can't play bridge anymore and...' she winced, 'and I can't even go shopping or for a short walk.'

'Have you been back to Mr Sinclair? Did he examine you?'

'Yes, three times. Each time he just takes more x-rays and says that nothing can be done and that I have to learn to live with the pain. Now the nurse won't give me any more painkillers – not that they helped much, and I am miserable; miserable enough to come back to you!' Despite her pain she had a twinkle in her eye. Many of my patients like to tease, and mostly it's fun. Fortunately she had brought her latest x-rays. I put them up on the viewing box. Sure enough the compression fracture had been bad, but it had healed, leaving a distorted and unstable back. I had misgivings about being able to help her. The picture wasn't good, but five years in practice had taught me well: examination first, then the diagnosis and prognosis, and only then a plan of action.

The long and the short of it, confirmed by a two-minute examination, was that the pain in her back wasn't coming from the fracture, but a good fifteen centimetres away in the sacro-iliac joint.[*] All the orthopaedic tests were positive: the Posterior Shear, Fabere, Yeomans, and the SI compression test, the lot. There was some residual tenderness at the fracture site but that wasn't what was troubling her.

By the sixth treatment, Mrs Boucher was improving and smiling again. I had used a very conservative form of treatment on the elderly lady. She had quite pronounced osteoporosis as had virtually all women of her age, but nothing that couldn't support a vigorous exercise programme, some cross friction on the muscles with active trigger points, and a very gentle Chiropractic adjustment. It was time to revisit our first consultation eighteen months ago.

---

[*] Joint in the pelvis.

'You were very cagey about how you fell, Mrs Boucher, when you first consulted me. Are you ready to tell me?'

There was a short silence. She was lying face down on my table, out of eye contact, a position where patients feel free to talk if you're willing to take the time. It was definitely worth it. 'The old bugger is dead now, so I suppose I can tell you,' she said. She squirmed as the cross friction on the Gluteus Medius muscle was quite painful. 'We remarried and he became a pest.'

'Remarried?' I exclaimed. 'Go on.'

'I divorced my husband when I was about fifty. He was being impossible so I just left him, but it meant Poverty Street for me. I had to find a place to rent, I lost his medical insurance and his pension. I had to buy furniture, but it was worth every cent.'

'Ah,' I said.

'Well, eventually I ended up in Olive Schreiner Home for women, and lo and behold he was across the road in Jan Smuts House for men. He was pretty miserable, and so was I, so I started visiting him occasionally. He was just as impossible as ever and our visits always ended up in an argument.'

'So?'

'Well, I decided to remarry him.'

'That's interesting. Was it for love or for money?'

'Oh, for his money to be sure! My medical bills had started adding up. My blood pressure was high, I had developed a nasty tremor in my hand so the doctor put me on some very expensive medicine for Parkinson's disease, and so I started thinking: *if we got married again I could go back on his medical aid and, when he died, get his pension.* We would go on living across the street from each other. I would visit him now and again, which I was doing anyway, we'd have another argument, and nothing much would change, except that I could then afford to pay your fees.' She gave a muffled laugh.

I couldn't help smiling, even though she couldn't see me, rather like people smile or scowl at each other when talking on the phone. 'Quite a schemer, eh! Did it work out?'

'Oh yes. He died about six months later, and I am still on his medical aid – just as well,' she added a little hotly, 'and now I get his pension too.'

It gets to be a problem. People retire but, with double digit inflation, if they live another twenty years, medical costs become prohibitive. 'But what's all this got to do with a fall in the night?' I asked.

She gave a little-girl giggle. 'We remarried last summer. It was particularly hot those nights so I liked to leave my windows open. Next I knew, he was coming across the road at about midnight, climbing through my window, and trying to sneak into my bed. "You're my wife, you know," he would say. 'Fancy that, with both of us in our eighties, him nearly ninety, in fact.'

'So?'

'So, I tied a long piece of string to the window, with pans and bells tied to it so that, when he came intruding, I would wake up and could shoo him away before he climbed in. Then one night I tripped over my own mantrap. I suppose you are going to say, "*Serves you right for marrying him!*"'

Oh, and why was Bernard Preston angry? Because Mr Sinclair obviously didn't examine his patient again after that first consultation. He must have been in a hurry, assuming that her pain originated from the old fracture. I could easily fall back into that rat race, I thought to myself, still unable to forget the rebuke from a patient: *conscientiousness is, mostly, what makes the difference between good and bad doctors.* If Mr Sinclair had taken a little extra time, he would have known that Mrs Boucher's pain wasn't coming from the site of the old fracture. I was sad that Jeremy Thomas had left for greener pastures. We could talk, without either of us taking umbrage but I wasn't so sure about this *Mr* Sinclair.

I could never cure Mrs Boucher. She went on consulting me once a month, mostly reasonably satisfied with her progress, and able to play her beloved bridge again, still complaining about the cost, of course, until she died quite suddenly, the way I would like to. I still think of her now and then, sad that I never made it to the funeral. The first I knew of her death was when she never arrived for her monthly consultation. Some patients you never forget.

Chapter Four

STROKE I

A good scare is worth more to a man than good advice.

Edgar Watson Howe

It's always irritating when a patient misses an appointment. When it's the first appointment on Monday morning, it's doubly irritating. Sally, my secretary, has a superstition that, when the first patient doesn't arrive, then the rest of the day will be chaotic. I have to admit that she has a point, but we are all allowed to be found wanting occasionally. It's part of life to be forgetful, or have the car not start on a winter's morning. It's not often though, that a patient misses the first appointment on a Monday morning because his wife was struck by lightning over the weekend. Golf clubs make good lightning conductors.

Sally brought me the news a few hours later, and I went over to Jerry's place after work. His kids had started arriving and I felt a bit awkward, said my piece and left. His daughter was talking about 'an act of God' and their sons were just shaking their heads and saying things like: 'shit happens'. So it does. They were a golfing family and all three children, now young adults, were *scratch* players which is no mean feat. I wondered: *Is golf a dangerous game? What are the statistics?*

Jerry finally made the missed appointment about ten days later. Sally had booked some extra time knowing we would talk. It was not easy comforting him after such a 'meaningless' death. A stroke of fate. On his way out, he said: 'One of the kids looked it up on the web – there's about a one in a million chance of being struck by lightning while playing a game of golf. Why did it have to be Sonia?' Why indeed?

I sat pondering those statistics that evening with Helen. 'One in a million. Just how dangerous is that?' I asked her.

'Do you mean: If you were a golfer what would the chance be of you being struck on the golf course this weekend? Struck by lightning, that is.' Helen, the mathematician, didn't need a calculator though she reached for a piece of paper and a pen.

'Yes, let's assume that the average player plays golf, say 25 times a year.'

'You go soaring far more than that!' she exclaimed.

'Nonsense! Once you add up rainy weekends, holidays and congresses then I bet it's no more than 25 times a year. I'll get out my gliding log book if you like.'

'Okay, okay,' she tried to placate me. 'Then if we work on forty years, probably a bit on the high side but nice for the figures, that comes to 1000 golf-days in a lifetime.'

'That means that, on average, one in a thousand regular golfers would be struck down by lightning on the golf course during their whole lifetime. A good deal safer than soaring or motorcycling don't you think?' I made a phone call. 'Shafton Golf club has about 500 members.'

'That means that, in eighty years, one person would be struck by lightning on the Shafton golf course, on average. I think I'll take up golf. It sounds like a pretty safe sport.' Helen was enjoying teasing me, knowing that she knew that I knew, that all she needed for peace of mind was a patch of earth. Her favourite saying was: 'When the world wearies, and Bernie ceases to satisfy, there's always the garden.'

'Of course, a second person could be struck next weekend.' I had to have the last word.

On average. So why Sonia? No one ever remembered another player being struck down at Shafton's golf club. Statistics. They can be useful. *Lies, damn lies and statistics,* my aunt used to quote, knowing how figures can be manipulated to prove a point. Still, I decided that one death in a million made golf indeed a very safe sport as far as lightning is concerned.

'One would probably more likely be hit on the head and killed by a mis-cued ball,' said Helen thoughtfully.

I agreed. No doubt, though, there would be less angry shaking of clubs at passing clouds, after a wicked hook shot dragged the ball into the thick rough.

It was not many weeks later that I was taking the history of a middle-aged woman during an initial consultation. She was a pleasant enough looking woman, and she shared with me the absolute misery of her headaches, ever since a fall off a horse in her childhood. Horses are dangerous animals, a lot more dangerous than lightning on a golf course, especially when crazy parents encourage their children to climb on some wild nag at a guest farm. She went on to tell me how at least once every six weeks she would go out of circulation for three days with the most awful pounding headache.

'Do you ever get nauseous, Mrs Anderson? Does it affect your vision?'

She nodded, confirming many of the classic migraine signs including nausea and occasional vomiting and, on occasion, all the stars and stripes, though jagged, of the American flag. Two or three days would be spent on her bed with the curtains pulled, in a drugged sleep. Could I help her?

'Well, I may be able to help you, Mrs Anderson. Chiropractic does help many people with migraines, but first I must examine you and find out if you have any signs of subluxations in your neck, whether you have active trigger points in spinal muscles or even perhaps a problem in your jaw joint. Is there anything else that may be important, which I haven't asked you about? Are you in good health, as far as you know?'

'Yes, I am in good health, other than these headaches. Once or twice when I have the headache, I find I can't think straight; a sort of muddled thinking,' she tried to explain. 'Once it was so bad I could barely speak intelligibly for an hour, but then it passed.'

'When was that?'

She thought for a few moments. 'Perhaps three months ago, maybe longer.'

'Did you consult your doctor?'

'Yes, he was quite concerned, and said if it happened again I would have to have some tests.' I nodded.

'Would you please go and change in that cubicle, strip down to your underwear and put on the gown, with the opening at the back.'

She came back in a few moments. 'I'm afraid I don't feel too well. I think I am going to be sick…' Her voice became a croak as she tried to force the words out. I sat watching, bewildered. What was happening? She tried to sit, missing the chair and fell to the floor, slumping to the side. As I watched her, the right side of her face started to sag and she grunted out a few inaudible sounds before collapsing to the floor, unconscious, all before I had laid a finger on her.

I rushed to the phone, and called the hospital. 'Please send an ambulance immediately to the Back and Headache Clinic in Chapel Street. This is an emergency!' I turned back to Mrs Anderson who was now lying on the floor. I took her pulse which was thready, but she was breathing, her eyes closed and her face now completely twisted in a grim mask on the right side. Suddenly her left arm gave a tremor, and she groaned, and I knew she was dying. There was absolutely no need to follow the three point test for a stroke. Could the patient:

speak intelligibly?
smile?
raise their arm?

Even a layperson could easily see all three were affected. I wondered whether I would have to start CPR and checked her pulse again. I could just feel the pulse in her neck, and leant down to hear if she was breathing. She was, though she was gasping and struggling for air. I loosened the gown from around her neck, relieved to hear the siren outside. Moments later Sally burst in: 'What's happening?'

I shouted: 'Bring in the paramedics. Quickly!' Mrs Anderson gave a little gasp and, when I felt again, there was no pulse, and nor was she breathing. I had never done mouth-to-mouth before on a real patient, and my mind raced. One, one thousand, two one thousand, three one thousand, was that it? I made a reluctant start, extending her neck and blocking her nose. Two burly men came rushing in, I could have kissed them but my lips were otherwise engaged at that moment. One quickly set up a drip and the other pulled out the cardiac massage machine while I went on for a moment longer, losing my rhythm. They took over very professionally, injecting her with something.

Mrs Anderson had died in front of me, before I had laid a finger on her. They managed to get her breathing again, and it wasn't more than a few moments, though it seemed like interminable hours, before they had loaded her onto a stretcher and carried her out to the waiting ambulance, still standing outside my office with lights flashing and a siren going. It wasn't the kind of advertising that a chiropractor would want outside his office.

That night I realized there were difficulties ahead. There would be those who said that I had manipulated her neck – which is what I was going to do, most likely, if I found subluxations and there were no contra-indicatory signs – and caused her stroke. There would be others who would accuse me of having treated a patient without having first examined her: my examination pad had only a detailed history, and nothing else.

I went early next morning to the hospital. Mrs Anderson was in a coma. Her daughter was sitting there, holding her hand and the doctor was doing his rounds. He was also my GP so I knew him quite well, not that I had the need to consult him too often, but Helen and the kids had certainly had their share of mumps and measles.

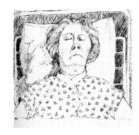

'Well, what happened, Bernie?' He wasn't his usual friendly self and Mrs Anderson's daughter scowled at me. I told him. He raised an eyebrow. I could read it all: *I'll believe you but thousands wouldn't.* He never said another word.

Mrs Anderson came out of the coma later that day, but she was horribly confused, and couldn't speak a word. After a week she went home, to the care of her daughter. I visited every few days. It was quite odd – Mrs Anderson was able to sing beautifully, songs that she obviously knew by heart but she couldn't utter an intelligible word. Five days later I arrived, and it was obvious that something had happened. There were several cars parked outside. The front door was open, so I slipped in quietly. Mrs Anderson's daughter was saying: 'I was holding her hand and telling her that John had got a hundred per cent for his mathematics test. Her eyes were alive and I could see she understood. She gave my hand a little squeeze, and then suddenly her eyes just went blank… and her hand went…' She gave a sob and wasn't able to finish, looking up for the first time, and seeing me. Her eyes hardened but she didn't say anything.

Next morning a burly policeman arrived a little after nine o'clock. I was busy with patients but he demanded to see me.

'Could you come back at ten o'clock, detective? Doctor Preston is busy with patients.'

'No, I cannot do that. I have my orders. I must speak to him now. Someone is dead.'

Other patients sitting in our reception rooms looked at each other. One leaned over and said: 'I heard that one of Doctor Preston's patients died here last week.'

'No!' the other man exclaimed. 'I wonder what happened?' he mused, looking at the officious policeman.

The first stood up. 'I can come back later,' he said. 'In fact, I'll just phone next week.' He left and the other man trooped out after him.

Just then I came through to collect my next patient. 'This man is a detective, Dr Preston. He needs to see you,' Sally said. 'Now,' she added rather ominously.

'Come through to my office, detective,' I said shaking hands with him and ushering him into the office where I did my initial consultations. It was in fact the same room where Mrs Anderson had died a few days previously, only to be resuscitated.

'There will be an inquest, doctor, concerning the death of Mrs Anderson? I have come to subpoena her file. Then you must make a statement and sign it.'

'May I make a copy of the file before you take it?'

'Yes, I suppose so. Would you make the copies now, please?'

I called Sally. 'Please will you bring Mrs Anderson's file. Make a copy of everything first,' I added.

After she brought the documents I put the copy in my drawer and gave the original to the policeman.

'Now will you please make a statement?' He passed me a sheet of paper.

I took my time. I knew my career hung in the balance. A woman was dead, and it was not entirely unreasonable to assume she had died because of something I had done to her. I was after all the last person to see her alive and normal. I wrote:

Mrs Anderson consulted me at 10am on Monday, 9th February, 2004. She told me of a long history of headaches since she had a fall off a horse as a child. She spoke of the severity of the symptoms, typical migraine signs that she had experienced, the previous treatment that she had had, and the medication she was taking, which included Migril and medication to prevent pregnancy. She was also a smoker of some 20 years and had controlled hypertension, so she said. She stated that it was 152/96 on her last consultation with her doctor. She reported that she had no serious illnesses, or injuries other than the fall off the horse. She described some typical symptoms of a so-called TIA (Temporary Ischemic Attack) some three months ago.

I instructed her to disrobe and put on a gown for the physical examination. On returning she declared that she felt unwell and nauseous and collapsed onto the floor. I had just started CPR when the paramedics arrived. I had not even begun the usual Chiropractic examination.

I did not treat Mrs Anderson in any way. Our only physical contact was a handshake whilst still in the waiting room and, of course, the CPR.

Had fate ordained that Mrs Anderson had her stroke an hour later…

Chapter Five

STROKE II

If you remember only one thing, Mike, remember this,' said the respected surgeon – a rare breed, to be sure but they do exist – 'you will never become a good surgeon, or a good doctor, until you have filled a whole graveyard with your mistakes.

Dr Michael Sparrow: Country Doctor,
Tales of a rural GP

The only patient that I came close to *stroking*,[*] and I may have indeed caused his stroke, was quite different. Barry was a beloved patient of many years. He was one of those people whom I cared a great deal about, and I believe the feeling was mutual. I had seen Barry through many an ordeal and had come to respect him deeply. Not because of who he was or what he had done, or not done for that matter, but because of how he suffered with such dignity in the hands of those of us who call ourselves healers.

Barry first consulted me with a routine case of lumbago, or low back pain, but there was another unrelated complication. Two clearly distinct conditions became evident during the examination. First, a *lumbar facet syndrome*[†] that was quite acute but which normally responds well to Chiropractic care. There were no neurological symptoms or

---

[*] A slang word used by chiropractors in the very rare incidence when a neck adjustment causes a stroke. (About 1/1 million manipulations.)

[†] There are three joints between each pair of lumbar vertebrae: the disc joint and two facet joints. All three can be injured, singly or together.

signs. Secondly, he clearly had advanced osteoarthritis in the hip on the same side.

'Doc, I have had this pain in my back for about three months. It just won't go away despite my doctor's treatment. Do you think you can help me?'

'I may be able to. Does it radiate into your leg?'

'Mm, not really, but does hurt here in the groin,' he said, pointing. 'Sometimes it shoots down to my knee.'

'Well, first I must examine you, Barry. Would you please strip down to your underwear?' I watched him as he undressed, noticing the difficulty he had leaning to the side, and the distinct limp so characteristic of a condition in the hip joint proper. I say hip joint 'proper' as the hip, like the shoulder, can mean many different things. Any condition of the pelvis, is often called 'my hip', but the true hip joint is where the leg joins the pelvis.

While he was changing I put up the x-rays that he had brought. They showed the usual degeneration of the lumbar spine, typical of a man nearly sixty years of age, but there was no view of the pelvis, or the hip.

The saying by the old chiropractor who had drilled it into his students, one of whom I was privileged to have been, concerned the importance of a good examination. It was to be re-lived that day. *If you don't look for it, you won't find it.* How true, and how often those words have echoed through my mind. *Look for it, Bernie.* Arthritis in the hip is simple to diagnose during a routine physical examination; that is, if you do a proper examination. The loss of internal rotation, adduction and flexion and the positive Fabere test were classical. Barry's doctor also didn't know that a lumbar facet syndrome is as treatable by a chiropractor as is a Strep throat by antibiotics. Our treatment is a lot safer, too, than the anti-inflammatory drugs that he had prescribed: research done by medical doctors in the United States has proved that they kill thousands of Americans each year.

The anti-inflammatory drugs fortunately didn't kill Barry. They just hadn't worked; but the stroke nearly did.

Barry had been a patient for over ten years when I came close to killing him. I saw him through several episodes of the facet syndrome. When he asked for advice about the hip that had progressed despite my care, I eventually encouraged him to have a total hip replacement.

It was some months before I saw him again. I was disturbed at the rather grey look in his face. 'How did the operation go, Barry?'

'Quite well at first, Doc. I was up and about after a few days and, once the pain of the operation was over, I was really much better. I could walk better and started sleeping well again.'

'And then?'

'My thigh started aching again.'

'Was it the same sort of pain as before the op?'

Barry made a strange mixture of shaking and nodding his head, trying to make up his mind. 'It is sort of the same, only it isn't in the groin now. It throbs here in my thigh which I don't think it did before,' he said rubbing his leg.

'Is your back sore?'

'It aches a bit sometimes, but I can bend and twist without any pain in the back. It's not like my usual sore back.'

'Slip your shirt and trousers off and let's take a look,' I said. The ranges of motion of Barry's back were good. As he had said, he could bend and move freely, and all the orthopaedic tests for the back were relatively normal. They are rarely completely normal in a man approaching seventy. He certainly had some subluxations in his sacro-iliac joint and the lower joints of the back, but were they causing the throbbing pain in his leg? I didn't think so. I put up his x-rays again on the viewing box, noting again the quite advanced degenerative changes in his lower back. *Well, maybe,* I thought. I checked again: he had no obvious subluxations higher up in the back that could be radiating pain to the front of the thigh.

'Barry, I am not totally sure but in my candid opinion, this pain in your leg isn't coming from your back. To be sure you need a few adjustments, but I advise you to make an appointment with your surgeon for a check up of that hip.'

Barry had his three adjustments and then it was some months before I heard from him again. By then he had searing pain in the thigh. He went on to tell me that the surgeon denied that it was anything to do with the hip, and that it must be coming from his back. What he now needed was a back operation. He had referred Barry to a neurosurgeon in Durban, who confirmed that he definitely had a pinched nerve in the back. That was the cause of the pain in his thigh.

'Bernie, are you really sure this pain isn't coming from my back? Both an orthopaedic surgeon and now a neurosurgeon agree that I must have a back operation.'

I went carefully over the examination again. He clearly did have a degenerated spine along with most other seventy year olds. He did have some pain in his back. But none of the spinal tests reproduced the pain in his thigh. All the spinal neurological tests were also negative but Barry couldn't walk more than fifty metres before he had to stop and sit.

'Barry, I can't say that I am absolutely sure, but in my opinion, your thigh pain has nothing to do with your back and everything to do with your hip. The pulses in your leg are normal so it's not vascular.'

'Well, what do I do? I can't go on like this?' Severe pain for nearly five months was taking its toll, and it was clearly getting worse, whilst all the doctors and a chiropractor practised their skills. Unskilfully.

I picked up the phone and dialled Jonathan's Hyde's number. 'This is Chiropractor Preston here, Nona,' I said. There was another Preston in town, so I always announced myself thus to Dr Hyde's secretary. 'Would you ask Jonathan to call me, please, when he has a free moment?'

'Certainly, Dr Preston. He is in theatre today; is it urgent?'

'No, not at all, Nona. Anytime in the next few days will do.' I didn't like to put pressure on our only neurosurgeon unnecessarily.

I was at work early next morning getting reports up to date when Jonathan Hyde called. 'Hi Bernie, what's up?'

'Good morning, Jonathan. Thanks for calling back so soon. I have a case of thigh pain that is baffling. Everybody is telling him that it is his back, but he has had a hip replacement, and I'm sure the pain is from his hip, not his back. Any thoughts?'

'A bone scan is the only way, Bernie. That will tell us.'

'Ah, thank you. Would you mind requisitioning one for him? These damn Medical Aids won't allow me to order it. They are quite happy to pay for an unnecessary back op, though!'

'No problem, Bernie. Would you mind writing a short report for me, including all his details.'

'Thanks, Jonathan. I owe you.'

'More tests! I just can't afford all these tests. I'm a pensioner, Doc,' said Barry when I phoned him.

'Then tell me what you think, Barry. Do you think this is your hip or your back?'

'Oh, my hip, without question.'

'Then go for the scan. Otherwise you may end up having an unnecessary back op and you will still have the pain in your hip. Dr Hyde is going to order it, so your Medical Aid will pay for most of it.'

The scan came back positive for the hip: an area of high activity around the pin going into the shaft of the femur. A careful study of the old x-rays confirmed it: there was a high likelihood of infection going down the pin into Barry's femur and the prosthesis was coming loose.

'This reminds me of that Giles cartoon, Bernie. The one where there are four doctors standing around a patient with their heads bowed, and one looks up and says: "Well, we've narrowed it down to one of four things!" Only this time one of them is a chiropractor! So what do I do?'

'Let's see if we can find you another orthopod in Durban, Barry. Mr Sinclair obviously has no further interest in your case.' I phoned another orthopaedic surgeon and made an appointment. Barry duly went off and had another hip operation, only six months after the first. Some people seem to attract misery. The second operation never introduced any nasty bugs into the bone – but the joint kept dislocating, causing Barry tremendous pain periodically, requiring another anaesthetic each time to reduce it. After the third dislocation in five months, this time whilst putting on a sock, I encouraged him to go back. He was by that stage *gatvol** of all doctors, except for one Bernard Preston, in whom he had great faith.

Then came that fateful day which shook his faith in all his doctors. 'Bernie, I've had pain in my calf for the last week.'

Chiropractors always get excited about pain in the leg. His back pain had always been on the left. His two hip operations, and the third in which they put in wedges to stop it dislocating, were on the left. Now he had left calf pain.

'Bend forwards Barry, backwards, sideways. Let me raise your leg. Any pain in the back or hip, or your leg?' Nothing to do with the hip or back seemed to reproduce his calf pain. I started some deep palpation of the calf itself. It was very tender. Perhaps slightly swollen, though I wasn't sure. A test for a strained calf muscle was positive. So was a test for a deep vein thrombosis.

---

* Had a guts-full of something (Afrikaans).

'Barry, I'm not sure. I think you had better see your doctor, this could be a *DVT*.'[*]

It was some nine months before I heard from Barry again. He phoned: 'Doc Bernie, I had a stroke a few months ago. I'm getting over it but I thought I would just let you know why you haven't seen me.'

'Gosh, I am sorry, Barry. How are you coping?'

'Pretty well. I am still having some difficulty with my hand, but otherwise I am fine.'

It was nearly a year after his stroke that Barry again consulted me. I had forgotten all about his calf, but I asked him about his hip and the stroke, and then went back to my case notes.

'Mmm, last time you were here you had pain in your calf. Did it get better?' He looked mystified, trying to recall the pain in his lower leg. 'And when did you have the stroke?' He gave me a confident date *three days before* our last consultation.

'That's impossible, Barry. You were here three days after that date, with the sore calf.'

'Well, it was around that time. I have obviously forgotten the exact day.'

It bothered me all day. Had I caused his stroke by palpating that thrombosis in his leg? Had his doctor added insult to injury by prodding further? Had he not gone to his doctor at all? I didn't want to know but, to be sure, I was a lot more careful with pain in the calf after that.

Can Chiropractic cause a stroke? Well, yes. Has Bernard ever stroked a patient? Well, maybe, but not by manipulating the neck. That's a lot safer than palpating a painful calf muscle! Safer than golf, too.

---

[*] A condition that affects the lower leg. Research on travellers proved that prolonged sitting in aircraft raises the risk.

'Bernie, my Doc says I mustn't let you adjust my neck. He says it could cause another stroke. Is that true?' Barry asked me one day.

'Yes, it is possible, Barry. Statistics show that somewhere between one in 800,000 – 10,000,000 neck manipulations cause a stroke, depending on whose statistics you believe.'

'Forgive me for asking, but...' he hesitated, 'did you adjust my neck that day I had the sore calf?'

'I'll have to check my case records, Barry. I can't remember.' I opened the notes, scanning them carefully, grateful that I always listed exactly which spinal adjustments I gave. 'Nope, Barry, I haven't adjusted your neck for over eighteen months. You didn't have any subluxations in your neck,' I finished, hoping he would believe me.

'One in a million. That's pretty safe, isn't it?'

'About the safest medical procedure I can think of, Barry.'

Chapter Six

DISTRACTED

On a wagon, bound for market,
There's a calf with a mournful eye.

All the winds are laughing...

                                        Bob Dylan.

History taking is one of those routine, important, yet often dull parts of every doctor's working life. Some say that, to the discerning doctor, a careful history yields eighty per cent of the information needed to make a correct diagnosis. It's mostly ordinary stuff, vital clues here and there, but every now and then I have a day when the history makes my eyes bulge and my hair stand on end.

'When did the pain in your back start again, Pat?' I asked.

Pat 'double g & t' Piggott[*] was an elderly farmer from one of the remoter parts of the province. His spread was tucked up against the Drakensberg range of mountains where he and his family had to contend with the real cold that descends on some parts of South Africa periodically, especially in August when the early Spring weather layers the highlands with a thick blanket of snow. Mr Piggott was a favourite patient, and not just because he brought me every year a beautiful *two-tooth lamb*[†] that had been slaughtered and hung on the farm. He was just one of those thoroughly decent people of the earth. Helen and I could easily taste the

---

[*] Reference: *Frog in My Throat.*
[†] Young sheep with the tenderness of lamb.

difference of his lambs, the meat was quite unlike that of the poor creatures stressed from a triple-decker truck ride, bumping its way to the abattoir along highways fogged with suffocating diesel, impatient drivers shaking their fists at one another; it was tender, un-feedlotted[*] and un-hormoned.

'Wee-ll, it was one of those very cold mornings when we were castrating the lambs,' he said in a slow, outback accent that hinted of a Scottish heritage and a leisurely manner of living that allowed time for the contemplation of life. A life unchoked by busyness. My old-fashioned clock is the real boss in my office: it chimes relentlessly, commandingly, demanding and reminding me that the next patient is due. *What is the meaning of this headlong rush through life?* A retired actress, watching me, once said: 'Remember, this is not a dress rehearsal, Dr Preston. This is the only performance.' I brushed aside the disturbing memories and envious thoughts, trying to concentrate on what the Piggotts were saying.

Jean, his ageing wife, with the wrinkled face and deep grey eyes, that I could compare to the snowy mountain sky rather than a summer's day, and pursed lips that matched Pat's, interrupted: 'He didn't tell you just how cold. It was minus fourteen those few nights. We lost over a dozen lambs.'

More images from one of the most disturbing short stories you will ever read interrupted my train of thought. Jack London's 'To build a fire'. Uninvited thoughts are one of the blessings that curse those who love to read. Never could anyone ever forget that chilling tale of a man challenging the real winter of the Canadian north, his spittle freezing with an explosive crackle before it reached the snow, signifying fifty degrees of Celsius frost.

'Was your back sore when you got up in the morning?' I turned back to Pat, dragging my mind back to the present.

---

[*] Practice of feeding animals high protein diets for quick weight gain.

'Nah, bit stiff but no pain. Forgot to do my exercises, though.' Pat grinned. Looking at his expression the word *sheepishly* flashed into my concentration. *Damn these disturbances*, I thought, looking at the shepherd. He had beaten me to my question. One of the mysteries of back pain is that even missing one or two days of early morning stretches can mean weeks of agony. I was interested in some new research indicating that the low back's 'muscle corset' is turned off at night and after prolonged sitting. Pat knew what was coming; we'd been along that road before. 'Keeps you in business, eh?' he laughed. 'Puts mutton on your table, eh? What's so bad about that? Gives us another chance to diddle the Taxman, eh?'

More distracting thoughts; back to the days when I had actively tried to barter goods of one sort or another for Chiropractic care, so I could evade the taxman, only to discover that, mostly, backs then wouldn't get better, and the blessings of my healing touch seemed to move elsewhere. But Pat was a very serious sheep trader, and tax evader, or was it avoider? My accountant was always lecturing me to keep that in mind, the one definitely illegal, the other just on the legal side of grey. Pat and I had had a long and very fruitful relationship. I fixed his back. He paid me in mutton. He was the exception that proved the rule.

'So what happened then?'

'Wee-ll, I went down to the lambs, with the boys, when it had warmed up a bit and we got on with the business of castrating them.' I winced. I suppose the thought of castration would be disturbing to any male. Pat belonged to a whole generation that called their black employees "boys and girls". Mostly there was nothing malicious about it. It concealed a genuine, if paternalistic, concern for their staff, but of course only a fool would today call an educated black man "boy". 'By lunch time, I had finished my six hundredth lamb, but after lunch I couldn't get out of the chair.'

'Did you sneeze? Do you have to lift the lambs?'

Jean snorted: 'Just you ask him how they do the nasty business. Just you ask him!' She said it with the sort of: 'just you wait Henry Higgins, just you wait' voice.

I wondered what was coming.

'Nah, you don't want to know the details of castration. It might upset you a bit. Wouldn't buy any more of my mutton, and then I'd have to pay you in real money, and you'd probably add VAT. Nah, I'm not telling you.'

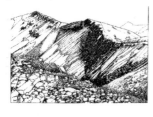 Although Pat had the sing-song voice of the mountains, his 'nah' sounded just like the nasal 'maa' of his sheep. The voice of a man who lived with yodels and sheep bells, and bleating sheep. You could only reach the Piggott farm from so-called civilisation by ox-wagon, horse or 4X4. Wild herds of Eland visited his pastures by night and Black Eagles probably took the occasional sickly lamb; a valley of fast flowing, trout-filled rivers and an infrequent hungry leopard.

Again, for just a moment I indulged in a half-musing, half of my mind listening intently to the Piggotts' story, whilst the other revisited my last Spring hike up to the Injasuti Peak; the bitter cold of Upper Cave with its tiny stream covered all day with thick ice.

I focussed again on the history, knowing that these thoughts would again endeavour to slip, uninvited, back into the present instead of behaving themselves by remaining in my dreams or a Sunday afternoon half-consciousness when it was appropriate. I never knew quite what to do with these unbidden images that, on the odd irritating day, caught me by surprise, slipping silently, almost like a spell from their subterranean world. That day was one of those days. I gave a little shake of my head, refocused my glassy eyes, quite sure I had only been gone for a quarter of a second, and found them both staring at me.

'Are you okay, Bernie? Did you lose us for a moment? You don't suffer from epilepsy do you?' I had been on a first name basis with the Piggotts for over twenty years and they knew me as well as any patient.

I blushed. 'Gosh, I'm sorry, Pat. That was naughty.'

'Penny for your thoughts,' piped up Jean. 'They looked interesting.'

'Two pennies,' said Pat.

'Are you going to pay?' I asked. 'How long was I gone, anyway?'

'Only three seconds, maximum,' said Jean, 'but I could see that you were far away.'

They were kind folk, trying to relieve me of the guilt that I was feeling. That was three seconds that they were paying for, and I might have missed a vital piece of the jig-saw puzzle. 'I'll tell you later when we're done here, and you've found your pennies. Now let me see, where were we? Ah yes, you were going to tell me about this castration business and how you hurt your back, Pat.'

It was Pat's turn to blush, and the shepherd again looked very sheepish.

'You have to bend over for a couple of hours while you're doing the business. The boy holds the little lamb on a table, with its knees tucked up like this.' He demonstrated and I well imagined a man holding a bundle under his arm pit, with both hands holding the back legs with the hips in the fully flexed position, exposing the poor thing's infant crown jewels. Pat had walked into my consulting room, leaning forward on a shooting stick. Any attempt to straighten up gave him a very sharp stab of pain down his leg. As he tried to demonstrate how the assistant held the lamb he gave a gasp, going white as he clutched his leg, falling back into the chair with a groan. He leaned forward again which gave him a measure of relief, beads of sweat pouring from his face. Ouch! Sciatica hurts. If he got relief bending forwards, then we were most likely dealing with a case of spinal stenosis, that term which strikes fear into the heart of many a chiropractor and patient, but what always surprised me was how few cases of stenosis I had to refer to Jonathan Hyde, Shafton's guru with the sharp knife.

As the spine ages, the disc narrows and a part of the vertebra called a *facet* starts poking into the foramen[*] from which the nerve root emerges. The facet degenerates with age and injury as it continually bumps the top of the foramen, beginning to curl forwards like a nasty tiny scimitar until it unerringly finds its intended victim, the nerve root.

I gave him a moment. It wasn't long before *his* eyes refocused on me and I knew he was ready to continue. A quick glance at Jean left me perplexed. Her eyes were swimming, but the corners of her normally pinched mouth were turned up. She didn't know whether to cry at her beloved of sixty-two years's pain, or to laugh at what was coming.

'Well, go on, Pat. Is there anything more I need to know? Sometimes the little details are important.' *Was the collision head-on? Were you facing the front? Did you have time to tighten your muscles? Did the car roll? Did you have pain immediately?* All these little details can sometimes reveal important information.

He glanced at his wife as she said: 'Go on, Pat. Tell him the whole story.' Jean brooked no alternative. *He also has a 'she who must be obeyed,'* I thought wryly, wondering what was to come.

Mind finally made up, Pat ploughed into the story, withholding nothing. 'Well, you've only got two hands, see. The poor little beggar is sitting on his bum, so to speak, giving little maa-maas. You know, how lambs do. The mothers are calling, 'cause you've just separated them from their little darlings for the first time and the whole shed is in an uproar. You take the knife in your right hand, give it a

---

[*] Hole where the nerve emerges from the spine.

quick run over the steel to give it a good edge, grab the scrotum with your left and cut off the end of the bag. I winced, not trusting myself to say anything and waited for him to go on. The tears in Jean's eyes began to glimmer with a sparkle, refracting the Spring sunshine, still pouring in through the bay-windows, giving tiny bursts of spectrum colours as she nodded her head approvingly, and the corners of her mouth were turned just a fraction higher. Gone was the pursed look.

'There's not much blood,' Pat went on, 'until you come to the tail but we'll leave that for a moment. Then you put the knife down, and with both hands squeeze the base of the little bag.'

I couldn't wait for the coup de gras. I could sense it was coming. 'And then?'

'You have to give a good squeeze – with both hands, remember – and then the two little knackers pop out.'

'Still connected, I presume,' I interrupted, thinking back of two long semesters in the human anatomy lab in Chicago.

He gave me an annoyed glance wanting, now that he was committed, to get it over as quickly as possible. I could see him thinking: *When is this stupid doctor going to shut up?* The poor old man's feelings were in a total muddle and I could see the prolonged sitting was causing him pain. 'Yes, still connected,' he whispered. 'If you let go with either hand the little beggars pop back in. So you do what shepherds have been doing for thousands of years. You grab each testicle in turn with the only implement at hand…' he stopped at that and thought for a moment, 'you grab each one with your teeth, pull it until the cord breaks off, spit it out, and then the other one. And then you cut off its tail and clip its ear,' he rushed on, finishing hurriedly. 'There! Now you know the whole sordid business of how I hurt my back.' Turning to Jean he said, not a little viciously: 'Satisfied?'

I was stunned but there was no doubt he was telling the truth. After the story had sunk in I said: 'You mean you bit off six hundred tiny lambs' testicles yesterday?'

'That's exactly what I mean, twelve hundred in total.' The tight look had returned to his mouth, but there was just a suggestion of merriment, mingled with pain, dancing around his face.

Piggott's Peak farm was an hour's drive, over the most atrocious roads, from Shafton. Since the first rule of Pat's treatment was that he was not to sit for at least a week, probably longer, and Jean did not drive, they came to stay with Helen and me for ten days while I worked on his back daily. Manipulation, or the Chiropractic adjustment as we call it, was risky for the first few days. He was in great pain, and there was considerable risk of the scimitar slicing into the swollen nerve. I used a series of stretching techniques, with traction and ice and my faithful Winks Green machine that gave alternating contraction and relaxation of the muscles. I even used a few needles. Many think the 'Winks' is just a muscle stimulator, but almost every muscle is attached at each end to a bone and I suspect each contraction gives a mobilization to the joint.

The first night we sat in the cool spring air on our veranda with a leg of lamb roasting gently in the kettle barbecue. Pat lay on an old *riempie** couch covered with cushions. Jean pulled out a little bag. 'I've brought you some delicacies for an hors d'oeuvres,' she said a little shyly. Helen turned up her nose when she saw the sheep tails still covered with wool.

'What do you do with those?' I asked, wondering stupidly if they could be used for tickling feet, like Helen feeling slightly revolted.

---

* Leather thong used for chairs and couches. (Afrikaans)

'Ha,' said Pat. 'Those are the best part of the sheep.' He started to struggle into a sitting position, but with a groan of pain sank back onto the couch.

'You stay right where you are, Mr Piggott,' Jean scolded him. 'Remember I've been roasting lambs' tails for over seventy years too. She took a tail in a pair of barbecue tongs and flamed it over the coals, burning off the wool. The smell was revolting. She dropped it onto the coals, reaching for the next tail. It was much shorter.

'Do some sheep have long tails and others short, Pat?'

He laughed. 'Naa,' he bleated. *How can a voice be both nasal and sing-song?* I thought. 'We cut the *hamel's** tails much longer so you can spot them.'

'How much longer?'

'Oh, about six inches compared to about one inch for the females.' His generation still thought in feet and inches, that archaic mode of measuring that our British forebears brought to South Africa, still used by certain backward nations and glider pilots. I had enjoyed teasing my friends in school in Chicago.

We sat quietly crunching the tails while Pat lay on his bed of pain, my Staffordshire Terrier waiting patiently at my feet for morsels. Later Pat had to perch on the edge of an old table with his feet on the ground, half sitting and half standing, to enjoy his dinner which Jean had sliced into mouth-sized morsels. The roasted onions wrapped in foil and the sweet potatoes with fresh green peas from the garden made for a meal that few anywhere in the world can better for taste or nutrition. Cloves of garlic and sprigs of rosemary carefully stuffed into the mutton gave off their aromatic scents and had us salivating like Pavlov's dogs. There was a small bowl of fiery red Inferno peppers sizzling gently in butter in a corner of the kettle. Mint sauce completed the meal. We weren't

---

* Male sheep (Afrikaans)

dessert eaters normally and in any case I'd already enjoyed more than enough calories.

After a few days of being conservative, Pat's back pain was a little easier, but any extension of his spine still produced severe, sudden, sharp, shooting pain down his right leg to the sole and outer edge of his foot. My favourite orthopaedic test called Slump 7 was still very strongly positive. I knew it was time for more incisive action.

'We're going to adjust your sacro-iliac joint today, Pat. Gently, very carefully, and if it doesn't move, that's okay, 'cause tomorrow it will.'

'I ought to trust you after all these years, but could it make it worse again? That was a fearful pain I had in my back last week.'

It was a reasonable question. *First, do no harm,* was Hippocrates' admonition to the medical fraternity and it included chiropractors. 'Yes, I'm afraid it could, Pat, but I've been at backs for a long time now, and I know yours, in particular, pretty well.'

He looked at me dubiously. 'Yes, but...' His words dwindled. We'd been over the territory several times in the last few days, and he knew that the pain in his leg wasn't improving with my conservative treatment. It wouldn't be long before the calf muscle started to waste. I am always concerned when patients have more pain in their leg than their back.

'There's danger in every form of treatment I'm afraid, Pat, and ours is no exception. It's still a good deal safer than what the surgeon will have in mind.'

His S.I., as we call it, must have been waiting to pop, it let off such a crack when I was just setting him up for the adjustment. It's not entirely clear in my non-academic mind why the sacro-iliac joint has such a profound effect on the lumbar spine, particularly at its lowest segment, the fifth lumbar vertebra. Early medical anatomists argued vehemently with the chiropractors of the day, saying that it was impossible for the sacro-iliac joint to 'click' but that's plain nonsense as every Chiropractic patient can testify. You *know* that the joint can click. A early Swiss chiropractor by the name of Illi did pioneering work for his time, at the forefront of anatomical research, proving just how much the joint can, and does, move. Today it is accepted by all that it is a fully moveable joint and recently a chiropractor was invited to lecture on the S.I. joint to the Spine Society of South Africa. For the benefit of all, especially the patient, much of the humbug has, fortunately, gone out of medical–Chiropractic relations.

From that day the leg pain began to abate and after two months of hard work, much on Pat's part as he faithfully stuck to the rehabilitation programme, his back and leg recovered completely. Fortunately he wouldn't have to rip out any more lambs' testicles until the next Spring.

'Pat,' I said to him on our final consultation, 'surely your colleagues don't all go through that macabre process of castrating their poor lambs?'

'No, they use a rubber ring that strangles the blood supply.'

'Then why don't you?' I was mystified.

'Firstly 'cause I think it's cruel, the poor little beggars are obviously in great pain for weeks while the scrotum and testes gangrene and eventually fall off. Ever been kicked there?' he looked at me questioning. 'Secondly, because it's bad business. My lambs lose far less weight and I get them to market a good few weeks before the other farmers when the prices are better.'

'Why are you so keen on the Piggott lambs, Bernie?' my secretary asked me a couple of weeks later. 'I know they taste good but is there another reason?' Sally had got one of the lambs.

'In the feed-lots, Sal, they pump them with protein for quicker weight gain. A researcher at the University of Western Cape called Veith did some interesting research on how high protein diets in feedlots weaken the legs of animals. It causes weak bones, oddly even though the calcium content is high.'

'Then why do you eat so much mutton, Bernie?' Sal liked to tease me.

'Ha, you know it takes us half a year to finish that lamb.'

'Do you think that vegetarians have stronger bones because of their low protein diet?' Sal went on.

'I'm not sure, but I do know that high protein diets are bad for sheep and bad for us. They weaken our bones and general health and so I prefer to eat meat that hasn't been feed-lotted. Ask any of those guys who aspire to be Mr Universe about the pain in their joints when they get older.'

That little episode cost the Piggotts two lambs and they threw in another one for the ten days' stay. I couldn't face any of it for a week or two which the family couldn't understand, but I wouldn't tell them why. Finally, of course, the smell of roasting mutton was too much for me, and I closed my heart to all the little lambs and their torment. I did ask Pat never to send us a male lamb again though. The card from the Piggotts that came with the lambs gave me again a renewed appreciation of the difference between a job and a vocation. Those who come to healers for succour are effusive when they know you have gone the extra mile.

Chapter Seven

ALL THE MEN SWOONED

A guidance counsellor who has made a fetish of security, or who has unwittingly surrendered his thinking to economic determinism, may steer a youth away from his dream of becoming a poet, an artist, a musician or any other of thousands of things, because it offers no security, it does not pay well, there are no vacancies, or it has no 'future'.

Henry M Wriston, President, Brown University.

All the men swooned. Sandy MacDonald had that effect on those of us from Mars. She walked onto the stage looking like a goddess and all the males in the audience fell into the lap of her seduction.

Every year we had a clinic outing to dinner and a show. I figured I owed it to my staff and, in any event, the Receiver of Revenue paid for nearly half of the cost. To my mind, good staff, well paid is what makes for successful business, and the odd evening out with their spouses was always fun anyway. The office manager had made the choice: dinner and 'Private Lives' with Sandy MacDonald in the lead role.

By day Sandy was a psychologist by profession and was as hard as nails. She didn't suffer fools gladly, particularly those whom she perceived as simpering, depressed females. 'Face the pain, get off your butt and live life.' Not many doctors referred her patients, which didn't bother her in the slightest. Sandy knew she was a goddess and her ego was entirely tied up with her success on the amateur stage.

I had to give it to Sandy, though – she had succeeded with a few of my patients where everyone else had failed. Of course, she had also put a few even deeper into the pit with her tough, no-nonsense approach. A good many women hated her, not only because of the effect on stage that she had on their menfolk, but because she treated depression harshly and without much compassion. For some it worked, but in her letter of thanks for the referral of John Sampson, Junior she made it quite plain that John Junior wasn't going to be one of them.

I walked down the long passage to my consulting room without the usual spring in my foot. I didn't notice the warm winter sun streaming in. It was another glorious twenty-five degree day in South Africa but I wasn't thinking about the weather. As I walk into my office my eyes usually sweep around the paintings, all originals done by patients and a few glossy photographs of gliders. I didn't give them a glance that day. Even the wood panelling that I had so lovingly crafted in my workshop was ignored. It was a beautiful room, perhaps as beautiful as any chiropractor's in the whole world, but I was worried and I roughly ignored my daily indulgence. When it comes to drugs, I'm beat.

I sat for a long time looking at the young man sitting in front of me. John Junior, in turn looked back. He was unkempt, in his mid twenties, with long straw-coloured hair and flat blue eyes. The eyes of an addict.

'You don't know what to do with me, do you?' he said.

'Mental telepathy must be one of your strengths.'

'Not at all. I have seen that look on many people's faces.'

John Junior had been a patient for over ten years. His dad had first asked me if I could help JJ with the pain in his shoulder. Actually the pain was in what we call the scapula – the shoulder blade – and came from a heavy electric lead guitar that hung over his shoulder for five or more hours every day. He had been a pimply school boy who spent all his spare hours – *every* spare hour – either making an unbelievably bad noise with his guitar (so his dad and the neighbours said) or writing music at the piano. His class teacher had called his parents in, telling them that JJ would, in all likelihood, fail his final matriculation exam. They wouldn't have been so critical – none of them, not the neighbours, nor his teachers, or his parents – had they known that John was destined to be the only millionaire on that street and the only millionaire ever to graduate from Graystone High, all before he turned twenty-one. A real millionaire, in pounds sterling.

In the early morning he could be found at the piano, quietly tapping out sequences of notes and jotting them down on bits of paper that lay all over his den, when most other boys his age were still fast asleep. John was untidy as well as a prodigy. He would then spend hours at the computer typing his melodies onto a computer program his parents had finally relented and bought him one Christmas. I still remembered the day when both John Senior and Wendy came to the clinic for consecutive treatments. They came in together, taking it in turns to sit on a stool while the other was being treated. Joint consultations work with most couples but it certainly didn't with the Sampsons.

'I really don't understand it,' Wendy said. 'JJ just wastes hours and hours on that damned piano.'

'And drives us crazy with the din on his guitar. He has the damn cheek to call what he plays music. Yes, that's what he does, he *plays* when a boy his age, nearly a man should be working.' John was angry.

'He has cost us an absolute fortune with his guitars and amplifiers, and computer programs and God knows whatever else.'

'It was *your* mother who got him started on the piano lessons. Remember she paid for the first six months and then left us to foot the bill for the next ten years,' he said accusingly. 'We would be rich, if it wasn't for JJ.' JJ's father was prone to gross exaggeration.

I might as well have not been present.

'Now they tell us he's going to fail matric. It doesn't surprise me actually; he doesn't do a scrap of work. He makes me so angry!' This Wendy said to me. She was lying on my table and I could feel the anger surging through her body under my hands. It came as no surprise that she was in knots. I suppose it was cathartic for them to get all that anger out but I resolved to treat them separately in future. They fed off each other's anger, and the bitterness was turning into a deep active *myofasciitis*[*] that made my treatment sessions very difficult. It raised an old question that always gets chiropractors arguing: *Do muscles in spasm cause subluxations of the spine? Or do subluxations cause muscle spasm?* Absurd, of course, because both are true.

John and Wendy were both lecturers at the University. True academics, John in the natural sciences and Wendy in mathematics, they could not understand how they had spawned a totally non-academic son. Their elder three children all went into university careers. But John Junior!

Actually JJ was very bright. In the last two weeks before his final high school exams he put away his musical instruments and put the same amount of energy into his school books as he did into his music and surprised everyone. He easily obtained a university entrance and an A for Mathematics. That unfortunately only made his troubles worse.

It's strange how one remembers conversations as though they had happened yesterday. John's parents managed to continue to have joint consultations with me despite my objections.

'There's no security in the arts,' Wendy said. I sighed, knowing where this conversation was going, knowing too

---

[*] A muscle condition in which the waste products of metabolism build up in the tissue.

that I was helpless to cut if off. 'He's not going to be a John Lennon or a Freddie Mercury.'

'You can be pleased about that. They both died long before their time!' I said, thinking how dated their knowledge of the modern music scene was. I suspected they had no idea that both Lennon and Mercury were dead.

'There's no future in music at all,' John Senior said, ignoring me. 'I can see we will be supporting him until we are old and grey.'

'Music makes a great mistress, but a lousy wife. He must go on and do a good solid degree.'

'But Wendy, isn't your daughter a lecturer in the fine arts department?' Finally I managed to get another word in.

'She and I are the exceptions that prove the rule. Very few women end up in the careers where they studied. They go and have babies and by the time they come back to the work place they usually do something quite different. Women should study their passion.'

'Yes, men must go into a career where they can provide for their families. There's no money in music. They just become bums and drug addicts.' John Senior was right in one respect.

I couldn't believe the blatant generalizations I was hearing. 'You mean young women can go into the careers they dream of, but men are not allowed to dream dreams? I think you two are amazingly sexist,' I went on, trying to make a joke of it.

No future, no security, no money. That's a musical career in a nutshell. How wrong they were. Perhaps they were unwittingly trying to steer their son away from a path in life that was to bring him – and them – much pain but their gaze into the crystal ball of life was very fuzzy. There were pots of money at the end of JJ's rainbow, a glorious career and a stunning wife. I couldn't see it either.

John and Wendy were utterly against their son continuing with a career in music. A Bachelor of Music degree at the university was out of the question. It was quite clear to them that the astonishing grade in Mathematics was where JJ's future lay, not realizing that math and music were more than just alliteration. If only JJ had obtained an ordinary D pass they would perhaps have left him in peace. Why couldn't he see it? Anybody who could get an A with the amount of commitment that JJ gave to his studies must be a natural: all his career-blind parents could see was a great future in Mathematics or one of the sciences.

I watched with sadness the deterioration of the family relationships as JJ's parents refused to pay for his musical studies. The knots in Wendy's neck grew worse and ultimately JJ packed his guitars and his computer and moved out. John and Wendy rarely heard from their son, an angry and hurt young man, though he kept in contact with his siblings. For some unknown reason, he also dropped me the occasional card.

Generally I avoid the Sunday newspapers. You can waste a whole day reading the week's Bad News. But a visitor had left the paper and I spent half an hour perusing the sports page. Just as I was about to toss it aside, John Junior's photo caught my eye in the Arts section. Long unkempt hair in dreadlocks, numerous rings and studs cluttered his ears and an unusual looking ring and chain connected his nose to his ear, caught my attention. I didn't like the dull look in his eyes but the paper was raving about South Africa's newest rage: The Larney Boys. They were destined for fame according to the writer.

Next morning Wendy was my first patient. 'You saw JJ's picture yesterday, I presume,' I opened the conversation.

'Yes,' she sighed. 'Didn't he look awful? I'm so ashamed of my son.'

'Why ashamed, Wendy? He apparently has a great future in music.'

'Bernie, you and I both know that for every thousand music groups, only one makes it to the Big Time. He's going down a cul-de-sac. He looked so awful with those rings and chains. And his hair!'

'Those are only the symbols of a youth that wants to do their own thing. That's their way of expressing their independence, Wendy.'

'I'm sorry, Bernie, John and I just don't share your optimism. I can only see him becoming a millstone around our necks and I'm terrified of him getting into the booze or drugs scene.'

'Well, that's true, but pushing him away from you is just going to make matters worse. He needs you, Wendy. It's time to mend some bridges.'

She just shook her head and never said another word during the remainder of the consultation. I did some painful cross-friction on a muscle in her neck and showed her how to do some new stretches that I had learnt at a sports congress. After adjusting two bones in her neck and another between her shoulder blades I dismissed her, sadly watching the strained, tense lady go on her way. I had a bad feeling about their family.

The Larney Boys did make it to the big time, amazingly quickly. A South African tour was quickly followed by their first CD release and then their first real break. A contract for a tour of England that smashed the records for the last decade of the twentieth century. John junior and his pals were rich. Very rich. That's when JJ's trouble really started: it is only to the very unfortunate that wealth and success come so early in life.

'JJ, you need help. I'm not telling you something you don't know. When you are ready I suggest you consult this psychologist,' I said, passing him Sandy McDonald's card. 'Don't be deceived by her pretty face,' I warned.

John junior turned over the card in his hands looking at it in a dull way – everything seemed to be going at half speed that morning. Finally he asked: 'Are you going to make the appointment for me?'

I thought about that. I had learnt the hard way that when parents and friends made appointments for others, they often don't arrive. Whilst I usually make the appointment when it comes to referrals, I quickly decided that it was important for JJ to have enough commitment to pick up the phone and make his own arrangements.

'I could, JJ, but I want you to make the appointment. She practises from home but her secretary will make the appointment for you. Shall we get on with the treatment of your back?'

My examination was a particular sadness for me. I hadn't treated him for some years. The huge bulging deltoid and forearm muscles that JJ showed off when he left school were wasting. Part of my treatment in those days had been a consultation with a biokineticist that led on to a gym contract. We had also designed a new strap that spread the load away from the muscles of the shoulder and neck. As JJ had started to work out, together with my spinal adjustments, finally the pain in his neck and shoulders from long hours hanging over his musical instruments had begun to abate. Just as important for the pimply teenager, the girls had started taking notice. JJ's ego had taken a battering from his parents and teachers but the combination of pumping iron and strumming guitars had begun to work its magic on the fairer sex. But now the increasing *kyphosis** of his mid-back and what we call 'disuse atrophy' of his muscles, coupled with the effect the drugs were having on his neurological system, was seriously depleting JJ's health.

---

* Viewed from the side the spine has three natural curves. In the midback it is called a kyphosis. In the neck and low back, a lordosis.

I treated JJ and, as a passing remark, said: 'Please also renew your contract at Andre's gym.'

JJ had come, despite his wealth, close to the gutter. He was fortunately wise enough to know it, and honest enough despite his drugged state not to lie to himself, even if he lied to everyone else about his drugs. Sandy McDonald's secretary was also a patient of mine. A few days later she said: 'I've never heard such a commotion! The shouting, and the swearing – you should have heard it!'

'It must be fun at your offices from time to time,' I said.

She smiled back: 'He left in a storm, but he did phone later in the day to make another appointment.'

Silently, I was pleased that the prodigal had come home. There was only one problem: in this case it was the prodigal's parents, not his brother, who were displeased with JJ's return.

Some weeks passed before I heard. John Senior's consultation for a severe headache, tension induced, brought back to me all the pain that this family seemed destined to experience. JJ was in hospital after an overdose. It was the season of good cheer, that time of the year when people are on holiday, without the pleasant distractions that work can bring. A season which brings many a family into crisis. It's no coincidence that suicides and family quarrels increase, and psychiatrists' consulting rooms are full at Christmas. During the rest of the year we can sweep the unpleasant stuff under the carpet.

John Senior was miserable. He didn't want to talk and I gave him space while I worked on his neck and shoulders. The muscles, it seemed, had been replaced by cords of steel causing serious fixations in the joints. Finally he said: 'We were so wrong about JJ. He has made more money by his 21st birthday than Wendy and I together will earn in our whole lives. Fat lot of good it's done him, mind you.'

'Have you told him?'

'Told him what?'

'What you have just told me. How wrong you were.'

'I couldn't! What would I say?'

'Just exactly what you said, without the last sentence about how little good it's done him.'

'What would that achieve?'

'What do you think?'

'I just couldn't, Bernie. I don't know what I think.'

I thought back to the days of my own children's youth: 'I remember the first time my son grasped something important that I couldn't understand, John, and how shocked I was. Actually I was quite angry, I'm not sure with whom. It took me several months to realize how pleased that Helen and I should have been that we had produced such an intelligent son.'

'Look, I know we really screwed up, Bernie. He's actually brilliant and we made him think he was dirt.'

'Keep talking John. You're on the right track, and any minute now you are going to add $2 + 2$ and finally get 4,' I said rather sarcastically.

'What do you mean?'

'I mean you are finally beginning to be honest with yourself. It's not my job to give you answers. You wouldn't like them anyway but when you work it out for yourself, then you will know how to deal with it.' I had been in the doctoring business long enough to know that folk have to reach that higher place themselves, the doctor's job is to ask the right questions, not give the answers. I suspected the only way JJ was going to recover was when his parents admitted to him that they had totally screwed up, hugged their very talented son and apologized for their meanness of spirit. Only then would JJ's ego begin the long climb back to feeling good about himself.

The call from Sandy McDonald was something of a surprise. 'Bernie, I haven't made any progress with JJ, but his parents are coming in, and you know I really think I see some movement in their lives. Ultimately that is probably where the healing has to come from. One day in the near future I am going to suggest to JJ that he go to a retreat for addicts called Shekinah. They do some good work there, but I will only put it to him once his parents have reached out to him. I think it's going to be soon.'

'What's your diagnosis, Sandy?'

'He's definitely psychotic. He has some bizarre false beliefs and, if you challenge him, he goes ballistic. He reacts so inappropriately.'

'I heard about the shouting! Sorry, I don't know too much about psychosis. Can it be caused by drugs?'

'Oh yes, absolutely, there's heaps of evidence. A very old study from Sweden on 50,000 army recruits showed that those who smoked marijuana had a six times greater chance of becoming schizophrenic. Quite a recent study by an epidemiologist from the Royal College of Surgeons showed that of those who smoked dagga only three times before they were 16, have a ten per cent chance of becoming psychotic.'

'Whew, that's high. I remember reading something about how safe dagga was. Safer than cigarettes.'

'Balderdash. You might want to read the latest *New Scientist*.* They spell out the research done, particularly how dangerous it is for those who start early with marijuana. Actually, we shouldn't write JJ off, though. It is the very young who are the worst affected and he didn't start until after he was 20, and there are some very good drugs today for the management of schizophrenia. His real danger is that he has also now started experimenting with hard drugs.'

'Is that what put him in hospital?'

'Yes,' she replied. 'I have achieved one small success though. One of his fixed, false beliefs is that he is a hopeless

---

* The more cannabis the young people smoked and the earlier they smoked it, the worse the risk of psychosis.

guitar player. Quite extraordinary. For two years he has denied himself his greatest gift, the very instrument that brought him so much joy. He was so passionate by all accounts.'

'No doubt about that. His parents told me he used to play for five or more hours every day.'

'Well, he has finally started playing again.'

It was some months before I bumped into a member of the Sampson family again. In fact it was JJ himself who came over and greeted Helen and me at the local Folk Music club. We liked to go occasionally. 'Hey, Doc, it's nice to see you here. I didn't know you were into this kind of music.'

I stood and shook his hand. 'You are looking really good JJ. Yes, Helen and I love music, and good guitar music is my own favourite. I'm so glad to see you've finally picked up your instrument again. How long has it been?'

'Nearly two years.'

'Take a seat with us. Can I buy you something to drink?'

'I'd love to but I'm up next. Can we chat afterwards?'

A girl with a sweet voice ended her piece, and then JJ went up onto the makeshift stage. 'Welcome back, JJ,' someone called. Everyone clapped and there were a few cheers and wolf-whistles. This was where JJ's musical career had begun some ten years before.

He started with an interesting fusion of Jazz and Classical guitar, and went on to sing a soulful song about a boy who had lost his way in the maze of life, until he finally came to himself. The small audience clapped and stomped their feet and his friends gathered around him; there was a lot of shoulder thumping and high fives. Later he came and sat with us.

'That was lovely, JJ,' Helen said. 'Bernie told me how talented you are. How right he is. That heavy rock CD you once gave us was not quite to my taste, but this was fantastic.'

He smiled at her and said nothing for a while. We listened to the next artist. Finally he said to me: 'That's quite a woman you sent me to. She gave me both barrels, and we had some real humdingers.' He winked.

'I am glad she could help. She's not everybody's favourite!'

'I can believe it! But she said something to me from which I just couldn't escape.'

'What was that?'

'Sandy said that either I had to face reality or reality would come staring at me in the face. It's not very nice when reality starts to deal with you. I couldn't escape her words, and finally started being honest with myself.'

'Did it come right quite quickly after that, JJ?' Helen asked.

He shook his head. 'Finally she said that she had completely failed with me and suggested I go to a retreat place for addicts. It took me a while to get there, but that's where I started facing the reality of my life for the first time in a long while. I realized for that I was literally going crazy and I could see it in those around me too.'

'So you managed to give up the drugs? Was that the big jumpstart to getting well again?'

He nodded. 'It was really tough giving up, but in the end I did it cold-turkey. I even gave up smoking. They encouraged us to plant strawberries, and pick Chinese guavas and make jellies and jams. In the end though I think what really made the difference was another guy at Shekinah. He had a delusion that he was a great guitarist, but he was hopeless. It so irritated me that finally I picked up his guitar and, for the first time in two years, started to play properly again.' He paused, listening to a new youngster on the makeshift stage. 'It was only then that I came to terms with my own delusion: that I was a hopeless guitarist and should never play again. I even started playing the drums, but there I really was hopeless.'

'Picking up your instrument was your way to getting well?' Helen enquired, intrigued.

JJ nodded. 'And you know what? Mom and Dad have been really good.'

'That's fantastic, JJ. Thank you for telling us. And now?'

'I'm not sure. I'm in no hurry, I don't need the money, so I thought I would start in this old jaunt for a couple of months, and I've been giving some guitar lessons to a few kids. I go out to Shekinah once a week for an afternoon, and help out, and well... I'm just happy to be for the present.'

A couple of months later we got the surprise of our lives. Helen and I were having dinner in a quiet steak house after a movie, when in walked JJ and Sandy – hand in hand. She wasn't much older than him, and that way (so she told me later) she was less likely to be a widow for ten years.

Chapter Eight

DANGER

In a perfect union the man and woman are like a strung bow. Who is to say whether the string bends the bow, or the bow tightens the string?

Cyril Connolly, critic and editor (1903–1974)

'Is gliding dangerous?' John Allsopp asked me one Tuesday morning. Whilst I am not pushy about soaring – not *everyone* needs to believe that it is the most spectacular pastime imaginable – I am always ready to talk to all and sundry. During consultations, over the last few months, John had been asking about the dramatic pictures that hung in my office: gliders soaring over Drakensberg peaks, or simply gently coming in to land at our airstrip. Finally I sensed the bug had bitten.

'No, gliding's not really dangerous.'

'What do you mean "not really"? When my son wrote off my car a few months back, and I asked him: "Had you been drinking?" he replied: "Not really"! What do you mean by "gliding is not really dangerous"?'

'Even if you climb up a ladder you'd better take care,' I answered evasively.

'Are people killed? Do pilots get hurt? Do they break legs?' John went on, irritated with me.

'Well, yes, sometimes pilots do get killed. Not very often but it does happen and, yes, occasionally they do break a leg. Usually both legs but mostly it's not very important because they break their necks at the same time,' I finished with a smile.

At this sobering piece of information I could see the light go out in John's eyes. 'The missus would never let me do it, then,' he said, sorrowfully.

I thought about that admission whilst I was measuring his apparent leg length, deciding how to adjust his pelvis. 'Does your wife wear the pants then?'

He too was silent for a while: 'Let's just say she wears her pants and I wear mine some of the time.'

'Just getting out of bed in the morning is dangerous, John,' I said. I decided the conversation was getting too personal, and changed tack: 'I did a good deal of reading and talking to pilots before I made the decision to go soaring. There is risk, but it's a measured risk mainly and, provided you use your common sense, soaring is not intrinsically dangerous. What finally clinched it for me was one Friday morning a patient never arrived for the first consultation of the day. Later his wife phoned to tell us that Tom had got up early and went out to mow the grass. There had been a heavy dew and he electrocuted himself. Like I said, just getting up in the morning can be dangerous.'

Saturday morning dawned bright and clear and after an early Bible reading and a quick prayer – too quick, I suppose, but it's always short on Saturday if the soaring looks good – I was packing my radio and lunch when John phoned: 'Doc, are you planning to go soaring today? Do you think Moira and I could join you?'

'That would be great, John. Be there by ten and bring a hat and plenty to drink. *Mad dogs and Englishmen*, you know.'[*]

Moira was an imposing lady. She stomped up and down with a sour look on her face, watching proceedings, and I had little doubt that she wore both her own pants and John's much of the time. Gliders took off, pulled by the mile-long

---

[*] Popular song made famous by legendary Noel Coward.

steel cable, with pupils taking their lessons early, and landing again five to ten minutes later. It all looked very routine and so it was. My turn came to drive the winch and I invited them to join me.

The launches were uneventful, the powerful V8 engine pulling the gliders high into the sky above our heads. They sat watching, John fascinated and Moira full of doubt.

'Who releases the cable?' she asked.

'When the glider is at about seventy degrees I cut the power on the winch and the pilot can immediately feel the loss of power. He then pulls the release cord.' They watched as I demonstrated, and we watched the heavy spring steel cable come tumbling out of the sky, with a small parachute attached so that it didn't bunch up.

'How high are the gliders when the pilots pull the release?' Moira again. She was asking all the questions.

'About fifteen hundred feet,[*] depending on the glider and the strength of the wind,' I replied. We watched as a small, light Ka8 struggled to find and then centralize in a weak thermal. Sharon was one of our more experienced pilots. Moira was watching, taking it all in; thinking too, by the look on her furrowed brow. Sharon climbed a bit, sank a bit, climbed again and finally succumbed to that great force of the universe, gravity. The day was young and the thermals were not quite strong enough yet, but I sensed that it wouldn't be long.

The ancient Toyota *bakkie*,[†] with nearly five hundred thousand kilometres on the odometer, arrived to tow the cable back to the launch point, out of sight over the crest of the hill. As fortune would have it, Santie, another lady pilot

---

[*] In a metricated world two measurements have escaped: the measurements of height and time. Throughout the flying world, altitude remains in feet. In this text we have included the height of mountains in feet.

[†] Small pick-up truck.

climbed out: 'This is the *relief of Ladysmith,*[*] Bernie,' she said with a smile.

'Ah, General Buller's aide, I presume. I never thought I would be thanking God for the English.' A lot of banter went on during those dull moments between flying. There were plenty of them. One of my favourite songs is: *I joined the navy to see the world, I saw the sea, I saw the sea.* There's a lot of sea between the magic flights that bring us out week by week, made palatable only by a good sense of humour.

John helped me load the small parachute onto the bakkie and hook the cable onto the *weak link.*[†] For just a moment I thought how the strategy of *The Weakest Link*[‡] was to blow the *strongest* competitor out of the sky. Somebody had decided to get Santie out of the way. She often took a club glider away to the Drakensberg for two or three hours while other club members pined on the ground.

The three of us squeezed into the front of the ancient cab. The doors were so rusty that the club mechanic had taken them off completely. Lovely in summer 'cause bakkies never came with aircon in the seventies. Only a Toyota would have survived the kind of battering it received at the airfield: all of our kids drove it whilst they were learning to fly. It was indeed ironic that they could get a flying licence at sixteen but had to wait until eighteen before they could legally drive solo on the road.

John was a mechanic by trade. 'You should contact the Toyota advertising department. They could shoot a documentary on this old workhorse, and maybe you could twist their arms for a new one in payment.'

'Yes, but they wouldn't give you one with an air conditioner,' Moira said with a smile. It was the first moment

---

[*] Famous English-Boer war siege.
[†] The weak link protects the winch if a knot hooks on the drum whilst towing out the cable.
[‡] Popular BBC programme.

of levity from her and I began to wonder at the formidable lady.

As we arrived at the launch point they were preparing for the first 'air experience flight' of the day. A burly sugar-cane farmer was giving his wife and small child a last hug, as though it would be *the* last hug and the duty pilot called out: 'Have you filled in the indemnity form, Jan?'

Moira pricked up her ears. 'Why do you have to sign that?'

'Just to protect the club if anything should go wrong,' called out the duty pilot. 'You sign all your worldly wealth over to the club in the event of a fatality.' The club chairman got mad at Dieter: when he was duty pilot he always had an amusing quip for prospective members – and every introductory flight is a prospective member. Not many people can walk away, untouched, from a flight in a glider. The chairman was afraid Dieter would frighten potential members away, but it never seemed to. What chased them away was the long discipline it took to become a safe and competent glider pilot. That licence didn't come cheap but the real cost was not measured in Rands and Cents but in the amount of life-force that had to be exchanged in acquiring it.

John and I went over to help with connecting the glider to the long cable. He bent over and I watched with interest as I saw his mechanic mind checking out the release mechanism. I did the 'back release' check – a safety device making the release from the cable doubly safe – and helped close the canopy. John and I couldn't help noticing the sweat pouring down the farmer's face. It had nothing to do with the African sun. We left the danger area and watched as the duty pilot gave the instructions to launch the glider. Out of sight over the ridge, the winch driver took up the slack in the cable and soon the great yellow bird, ungainly on the ground, climbed majestically into the blue sky. Small clouds were bursting out high above us. It was going to be a great day.

'Any more introductory flights?' the duty pilot called out, as they trundled the other club double-seater onto the launch point. John looked dubiously at Moira and I watched with interest, out of the corner of my eye, as the family contest played itself out. Was John going to get permission from Moira to fly?

'Yes, I would like a flight,' Moira called out. John was astonished. So was I.

'That's good,' called the duty pilot. 'Come and sign here please and pay your dues. Bernie, would you like to take this lady up?'

I balked. This was not how I had planned the day and it was definitely not panning out the way I wanted. Nervously I answered: 'Yes, okay. Help Moira into the glider, please John.'

I changed my broad-brimmed leather hat for a much smaller cap that gave me good all-round vision. Several gliders vying in the same thermal could be dangerous if they couldn't see each other clearly. By the time I got to the glider, an elderly Ka7 glider built in the sixties by a German company called Schleicher, Moira had already seated her ample frame in the back seat. I leaned over her, tightening the straps and pointing out the instruments to her. We always treat these flips as a first instructional flight. 'This is the ASI, Moira, or "air speed indicator". It's just a speedometer.'

'Then why not call it a speedometer?' she asked abrasively.

I winced, realizing this was going to be a difficult flight and wondering if I should ask one of the other pilots to take her up. Too late, I mused ruefully, a decision I was going to regret shortly.

'The ASI measures the speed relative to the air, and to that you have to add the velocity of the wind relative to the ground to get your actual speed.'

'Velocity? What's that?'

'We're getting too technical, Moira! Do you want to fly or do you want a maths lesson? Velocity is the vector quantity of speed, it has direction as well as magnitude. The wind might be blowing against you or with you, or in any direction for that matter.'

'Can't add scalars and vectors,' said Dick, the co-owner of my small Ka6 glider. He was waiting to hook the cable onto the glider. Dick was a lecturer in mathematics at the local University, and he couldn't stand me breaking a cardinal rule. We were good friends but enjoyed pulling each other's legs.

I scowled at him. 'Let's just call it an ASI, Moira. You will notice that we launch at about ninety kilometres per hour.' I went on quickly wanting no more awkward mathematical questions: 'This is the Variometer. It tells us whether we are in rising or sinking air.'

'Is that also a vector?' she asked.

I was exasperated, but realized it was not an unreasonable question. I hadn't thought about it before. Dick raised an eyebrow with a cheeky grin. 'Well, yes, I suppose it is, as it is positive when you are rising, and negative when you are sinking.' I sped on before she could pose another question: 'This is the airbrake,' I demonstrated, pulling out the lever and gesturing towards the airbrakes that protrude out of the wings. I wanted to move on quickly but, before I could take in a breath, Moira had again beaten me to the draw.

'Do they slow the glider down?'

'Damn it all, Moira, do you want to fly with me, or do you want a lesson in mathematics, aerodynamics and rocket science?' I had lost my cool and should have stepped away right then and there. 'There are other people waiting to fly the glider and this is not the time or the place for all these questions.'

For an aircraft to crash it usually requires more than one thing to go wrong. Often a string of blunders, and then some bad luck tacked on. We didn't actually crash that day, but it came close.

Quickly I checked that Moira was tucked in snugly and without another word, strapped myself into the front seat. Quickly I went through all my checks and the CB routine. Cable break. Instant decisions have to be made if the cable breaks. About the only thing that didn't go wrong that day was a low-level cable break. Another glider called in on the radio that he was on the downwind leg of his landing pattern so I snapped home the canopy and signalled to Dick to hook on the cable. Someone else rushed to the wing-tip and I prepared to launch, asking the question: 'All clear above, behind and ahead?' We had added the 'ahead' after my accident several years previously in my beloved Ka6.[*] The wing-walker looked up at the glider on finals. It was about to land. He shook his head: 'Abort the launch.' If there was time we usually rushed it with a shout of 'expedite' but I knew today was not the day. Apart from anything else I needed time to simmer down. I pulled the yellow release knob (just in case the landing glider snagged the cable that was lying on the runway) and opened the canopy.

'Why aren't we taking off?' Moira demanded from the back seat. Just then the landing glider whooshed about fifty feet above our heads, landing right in front of us. I ignored her question; she had her answer.

We sat for nearly fifteen minutes while the glider was retrieved from the runway and towed all the way back to the launch point. The instructor normally gives his critique the moment he and the pupil land and they were fortunately none too quick. Moira and I sat in silence, still strapped into the glider. By the time we were ready to launch I had recovered my equilibrium. I went through the pre-launch routine a second time, ignoring Moira's questions. I had never before refused to take up a passenger but I too was on a learning

---

[*] Reference: *Frog in My Throat.*

curve that day. I should have, there was drama to come. Finally, I was about to close the canopy, when a strong gust of wind came bursting through. It rocked the glider and I looked up at the wind sock to gauge the strength and direction of the gust. 'Just wait a moment,' I said to Dick. 'Let's see what's going to happen.' The gust died down but then another came through, less strongly.

'Just a thermal,' called the wing-walker.

You can feel thermals on the ground – they are just sudden movements of air as the air heats up and starts to move. Normally it's a good omen. You then often launch straight into the thermal and a good flight is assured. I nodded and closed the canopy and Dick hooked on the cable. We again went through the 'above, behind and ahead' routine and, after a quick glance at the wind-sock, I lifted my finger indicating to the duty pilot that we were ready to launch. One finger signals that the winch driver should take up the slack in the cable. Two fingers doesn't mean anything vulgar: it just means that he can turn on full power. The wind was a bit gusty for my liking, but not dangerously strong. 'It's only a nice thermal,' called Dick.

It wasn't a nice thermal. They were the first gusts of a southerly gale that was about to come bursting through. On the launch we were instantly climbing very steeply as the gale increased in strength. I signalled desperately to the winch driver, by thrusting full alternate left and right rudder. I realized we were launching much too fast as the ASI rapidly zoomed above one hundred and twenty kilometres per hour. Fortunately Santie, still on the winch, was ready for my signal and quickly cut back on the power. Anything a man can do, a woman can do just as well. Often better. Santie came from that pioneering Afrikaner stock where a woman had to be able to do everything that her man could do. She was one of our best all-round club members. She could even hold her beer a good deal better than many of the men.

We were launching at the limits. When another strong gust hit us the cable broke under the load with a loud 'ping' and the nose of the glider jerked up into a very dangerous attitude. We would stall in seconds if I didn't act quickly. Hours and hours of long training bore fruit as I pushed the stick forward, gently at first, and then more firmly as we were still nose high.

'What happened? What's happening?' came a cry from the back seat. The negative G if the cable breaks always brings an anxious moment to the novice. I could feel Moira's hand on the dual stick as she tried to take control, but having no idea what to do.

'Leave the controls alone,' I shouted, 'or you will kill us both.' The variometer was signalling strong lift in the frontal conditions and I had to make a snap decision. The cable had broken when we were seven hundred feet above the ground, so it was quite safe to make a few turns but I wasn't sure that I wanted to fly with the mad woman in the back seat. 'Do you want to fly Moira, or shall we land?'

'Is it safe? What was that jerk?'

'Just answer my question, Moira. Do you want to land? If you want to fly then you had better shut up and keep your hands off the controls.' I should have landed, no question about it, and I already rued the decision to fly with her. I banked the glider steeply whilst I waited for her answer. I also needed to know how she would handle the steep bank needed to stay in a thermal. There was no reply so I just kept the bank on. We were going up like a rocket as the cold frontal air undercut the warm moist air and variometer was banging against the stop at five metres per second of lift. Not a squeak emanated from the back seat. As we climbed I couldn't help noticing that we were also being carried far downwind by the gale. First, we were carried over the tall maize silos, about five kilometres north of the airfield, then Lake Msimang, and still we were climbing. It became very quiet in the glider and then it dawned on me that we weren't in a thermal. We were in 'wave'.

When a strong wind hits a sheer mountain like the Drakensberg, the air rises abruptly and then on the far side of the mountain it goes into a series of sine-wave type configurations. Very strong lift, even to tens of thousands of feet on the upside, and very strong sink on the downside. In between, where the sharply rising and sinking air abut, there is powerful 'rotor' that can smash a glider in seconds. We were in the lift, reaching ten thousand feet above sea level in not much more than five minutes. There was not a chirp from Moira and for the first time since the launch I began to relax. In this kind of lift I was not concerned at being blown down-wind. We could always get back from this height. Well, nearly always.

Then we hit the rotor. I had read about rotor but never experienced it. The turbulence was shocking. First the left wing was violently thrown up and the glider turned suddenly, then the nose was forced down sharply and we were diving and then everything was reversed with the glider on the verge of stalling. I don't know how long it lasted, losing all sense of time and position, just struggling manfully to keep us alive.

Should I radio the airfield? The words of our senior instructor came forcefully into my mind. 'Aviate, navigate, and only then communicate.' Thank God for Ainslee. He had soared since he was boy and then spent thirty years flying as a commander with British Airways. His wise words came back time and again to me in crises. Just then I heard a gurgling sound and then the unmistakable smell of vomit. 'Try to keep it in your shirt,' I called, feeling a little nauseous myself.

The rotor ended, just as suddenly as it had started. The air was silky smooth again – but this time we were sinking just as fast as we had climbed. I looked around and realized that I had lost five long minutes. I could recollect almost nothing, except trying to keep the glider flying. We had by now been blown far down-wind and, to get back to the airfield, we would have to fly back through the rotor. I looked around desperate for landmarks and with a sigh of relief found that we were just a little east of Lammergeier Castle and, nestled below it, Lake Pastel where we had spent so many happy hours at our trout-fishing resort. Some soul-searching hours, too. River's Bend gliding club was only ten kilometres away, further downwind and, twenty minutes later, I duly landed without any further to-do, heaving a sigh of relief. Moira never said another word.

I never heard from the Allsopps for some months. Dismantling the glider and packing it onto the trailer had been laborious and it was long after dark by the time we had schlepped it back to our club. It had been an exhausting and frightening day and I never really expected to see either of them ever again. Shocking and scary flights like the one Moira and I had experienced together were rare. Mostly they chased people far from soaring, but for me, I realized, it was what brought me back week after week. A little wiser, and certainly more experienced.

Then John made another appointment. He had hurt himself again. This time he had strained the capsule of his shoulder joint while trying to lift a heavy briefcase off the back seat of his car. After I had finished examining him, adjusting the joint with my little Thuli drop-piece and giving him a set of rehabilitative exercises, John asked: 'Doc, are there any good books on soaring? You know, the introductory types.'

I sat looking at John for a long moment. 'Yes, there are. There's a good one by a fellow called Piggott that I could lend you. What will Moira think?'

John just smiled and I agreed at first to bring my book to the office, before changing my mind. 'If you really are going to get into soaring, then you should buy the book, John. It's a standard reference for every glider pilot.' I knew how much work it took to write a book and I was going to make sure Piggott got his fee. More important it demanded that the Allsopps had enough commitment to find and order the book themselves. Those were the days before Amazon.com.

A few more months went by and then an astonishing day. Moira and John arrived unannounced at the club and both signed up as new members. 'Thank you for the book you suggested, Bernie. We both read it several times from cover to cover. You remember that flight we had together? It was the most delicious experience that I have ever had,' said Moira.

I watched with interest over the months how John became more assertive. He proved to be a natural pilot and, with his technical skills, he soon made himself invaluable at the club. Moira was her usual aggressive self and it wasn't many months before she was ordering other pilots around: 'Dick, it's your turn on the winch. Bernie will you fetch the cables…'

Santie cornered me one day in the bar after the gliders were all neatly hangared for another week. Gesturing at the Allsopps she said: 'It was you who introduced them to the club wasn't it, Bernie?'

I nodded, knowing that Santie had something on her mind.

'We're lucky to have them. The winch gives much less trouble since John took over the maintenance.'

I nodded. 'True. I'm glad I'm not married to his wife, though!'

'Oh nonsense, Bernie. Good marriages are a forty-nine/fifty-one per cent arrangement with the wise man giving way in areas where the good wife clearly has the skills and authority.'

'Yes, but…' I started.

'No buts. If the weak man is unable to take the lead when he is in *his* element then he mustn't complain if his wife always gives the casting vote. *Somebody* has to lead.'

I nodded vaguely. 'I must admit she makes an excellent duty pilot. Things always run smoothly when she is organizing the day.'

'Exactly.' We finished our beers.

A lot of pilots, particularly the men, were irritated by her, but Moira went on to take a leading role in the club affairs. John went solo after fifty-five flights, a good two months before Moira, and it did wonders for his ego. I watched him grow into the man I knew he wanted to be and, while Moira still ordered him around, as she did to most of the club members, John ceased to be the doormat that he had become. I noticed how he learnt to stand up to her and take his rightful place both at the soaring club and, I presumed, in their home.

Soaring has that effect on people. It is a dangerous sport and people do die occasionally but members learn to take responsibility and initiative and their children grow up very quickly in the gliding environment where they are treated like adults, each with their important roles. With few exceptions those children who become glider pilots grow up to take significant leadership roles during their adult lives. Enough said.

Chapter Nine

BERNIE GOES TO AMERICA

Large multicentre trials supported by the British Medical Research Council and published by the British Medical Journal have reported that Chiropractic management and skilled manipulation are more effective and cost-effective than usual or best medical care.

Brit Med J 300:1431

The queue for the toilet wasn't long but just long enough to get me thinking; from thirty-five thousand feet, in the middle of the long night, I couldn't even see a twinkle on the ground. For a moment I wondered who first called it 'darkest Africa'.

A young man looked over my shoulder, also waiting patiently, quietly murmured: 'Must be over the Sahara. No sign of life.'

Bored with looking at the dark night, unmoved this time by the stars which, in sharp contrast to dark Africa, filled the sky, my attention was drawn to the man in the nearest seat. He was fast asleep, snoring quietly, his head and neck hanging at the strangest angle. *He is going to be in pain in the morning*, I thought. Then my eyes slid to his neighbour. The woman was also fast asleep, faint smiles flickering around her lips, no doubt as she dreamed of the loved ones she would soon be seeing, her neck gradually slumping forward, down and down until it was in full flexion, but also twisted to the side; her head spasmed upwards, still deep in the arms of Morpheus, again beginning its jerky traverse forwards.

I heard the toilet flush and the door opened as a young boy made his way back to his seat. When I emerged I couldn't help looking at the other people around. *No wonder I am consulted by so many people after long trips*, I thought, irritated with myself – I was supposed to be on holiday, not pondering about stiff necks and strange postures on large passenger aircraft at thirty plus thousand feet in the middle of the night.

Later reflecting on my own breakdown, I wondered how many patients I had instructed to take a three-week vacation every year. The first week is spent getting the mind into neutral. Yesterday I was still in the office, and today, on my way to celebrate my father's seventieth birthday in New Hampshire, I realized I was still in overdrive, unable to drag my mind away from analysing the sleeping bodies around me, and a few patients in crisis that I had left to my colleague. A few passengers were reading or watching a movie but, for many, there was going to be pain in the morning. Maybe just a headache for a few days caused by an over stretched muscle, but for some much worse with subluxations of the spine that could cause neck pain for months. Less certain was the possible, even probable, effect these subluxations might cause to their general health, inhibiting that vitality that surges forth from the brain to every cell in the body. It wasn't going to be long before I was to find out how a muscle starved of that neuronal input would begin to ache and atrophy.

The seats were so uncomfortable that I couldn't sleep and my mind drifted back to a research dissertation I was supervising at the Chiropractic College. *Would the group receiving spinal adjustments respond as well as the group being treated with anti-inflammatories and an adjustment? Research? Damn! Why can't I turn my mind off?* I started turning over the idea of a dissertation on the sleeping posture in jets. Were all travellers prone to spinal pain after long flights, or only those who travelled at night and slept in these strange positions? I wondered if Atlantic Airlines would sponsor the project or if they would see it as a threat? On the negative side passengers might view the research as a comment on AA's seats – which it was – but all the airlines I had flown in had bad seats. In fact, AA had the best on that trip. On the positive side, they might be seen as a progressive airline, concerned about their passenger's health and welfare. I decided to scan the net when I got home to see how the research group got the nod.

Gradually it started getting light and I looked from my window seat down at the emerging dawn. There were dark shadows on the ground and a pink horizon with beautiful shades of grey, turning to pearly blue. The Mediterranean coastline came abruptly into view. *Algeria or Morocco?* I wondered, switching the on-board TV to the map of our progress. The cabin crew started offering cups of hot coffee and I took a deep breath, making a conscious effort to get into holiday mode. I felt myself beginning to relax as the hot black liquid warmed my innards, and I began to wonder how I would possibly get through the three hours at Heathrow before the second leg of the Atlantic Airlines flight left for New York's Kennedy airport.

Fortunately we didn't have to change terminals but I was bored and went into a bookstore looking for something relaxing. A Louis de Berniere about the cocaine trade in South America caught my eye. That would be right up my street, I thought, looking forward to one of my favourite authors. How wrong you can be, choosing a book from the cover and even the author. Select the right book for your mood, I realized later. I should at least have read the blurb on the fly-cover. It was a horror story but still I couldn't put it down, drawn on by the author's captivating tale. In any event it did take my mind off health: right into the grotesque realm of death.

Nevertheless, standing in the boarding queue for New York, I watched a man with his arm stretched over his head.

He was obviously in great pain and, simply from his posture, I made the diagnosis. I knew I wasn't wrong, though there were other possible causes of a pinched nerve in the neck. I recognized him as we had briefly chatted at Johannesburg International just prior to the long flight to Europe. The so-called Shoulder Abduction Relief sign, or SAR, was strongly indicative of a nerve root entrapment, and a serious one at that. I turned my mind back to the opium trade, wondering if a Chiropractic adjustment or a shot of morphine would be more effective for the seven hours it would take to cross the Atlantic. I had no doubts which would be more effective in the long term: that which treated the cause.

The pilot's call soon after take-off further disturbed my peace. 'This is your Captain. My apologies for disturbing you. If there is a doctor on board who can help a man with pain down his arm would they please contact a stewardess urgently.' My heart sank. *My holiday, my soul, my peace of mind.* I knew exactly which passenger it was. Finally, 'I care' won, and I turned on the light to call an air hostess. 'Has anyone come forward to help your patient?' I enquired.

'Yes, there is a doctor, helping him,' she replied.

'Thank goodness,' I said, stretching out in my seat. 'Would you please bring me a beer?'

'There is a doctor but the man with the sore neck is asking for a chiropractor or physiotherapist. You aren't... she hesitated... by any chance...?' She left the sentence unended, enquiringly.

'Oh, no! Are you sure?' What a fool. Of course she was sure. Reluctantly I dragged myself out of my chair, apologising as I stood on the toes of the man in the aisle seat. She led me forwards to a small private area where the patient was lying on a couch, with a middle-aged man in an open neck shirt checking his heartbeat with a stethoscope. I was impressed – he had brought the tools of his trade with him. Perhaps he was going to a congress. Mine were in far-off Shafton, hoping that out of sight meant out of mind but it was not so easy to escape the world and its demands: I hadn't left my hands behind.

'I think he is having a myocardial infarction,' the doctor said to me. 'He has pain down his left arm.'

'Are you sure?' I asked. 'There are other conditions that cause pain in the left arm.' It was indeed the same man I had seen with the SAR sign.

'Like what?' he snapped, staring at me. He may have had no idea I was a chiropractor, or perhaps he had guessed, but his aggression rankled me.

'Try the ranges of motion of the arm, do a brachial tension test, perhaps Speed's test, and have you checked the radial pulse?' That shut him up. He'd probably never heard of a Speed's test but at least he took the pulse. 'It's quite normal,' he said 'the same as the carotid pulse.'

I reminded myself that this was no place for rivalry. We had a patient in pain and he should be the focus of our attention. I asked the man: 'Are you feeling nauseous or sweaty? Have you ever had high blood pressure? Do you have a sore neck or shoulder?'

'My neck is very sore,' the man said. 'It started early this morning on the flight from Johannesburg.'

'Would you like to check his cervical ranges of motion and do a brachial tension test?' I suggested to the doctor who was still in the position to examine the patient. He looked at me hesitantly, *probably not unlike how I would feel if asked to palpate an ovarian cyst,* I thought to myself. 'Here, let me help,' I said giving him a warm smile. I was determined not to get into an argument. I turned the man's head to the left and did a few orthopaedic tests and it wasn't long before we had established the cause of his pain. A deep breath didn't affect the pulse in his arm, ruling out various possibilities. As soon as I stretched out the plexus of nerves that ran down his arm he flinched. That was why placing the arm over his head relieved the pain – it did the exact opposite, releasing the stretch on the nerve root.

'Hmm, looks like a nerve root entrapment syndrome,' I said using medical jargon. It hadn't taken me long as a young chiropractor to learn that giving a condition a medical and especially a Latin-sounding name made it sound far more serious. *Lumbago* just means *sore back* in Latin, *nerve root entrapment* just means a *pinched nerve*. Medicine does it all the time and we in the Chiropractic profession had learnt to play the game. 'Do you have any anti-inflammatories to give him? I'll leave you to inject him.' Turning to the hostess I said: 'It's important he lie down for the rest of the flight. I'll come and stretch out his neck if he's still in pain after the injection.' I returned to my seat, after thanking the GP, silently wishing him luck: Our patient was in a lot of pain. In my experience medication wouldn't even touch the deep gnawing ache in the arm of this exceptionally painful condition but, since one adjustment of his neck was not likely to bring much relief either, I had no desire to adjust his neck.

I had tired of the horrors of cocaine and turned to an old favourite Julia Roberts film. I had missed most of the movie but got really excited when I saw the actor, to whom I had once assigned the 'most irritating English actor of all time' award, reading *Captain Corelli's Mandolin* on a park bench with a very pregnant Julia lying with her head on his lap. The cover was unmistakable. I had chosen that book too (another de Berniere) on the basis of the cover alone. *If ever I take to writing,* I thought, *I must remember the sheer power of a glorious cover.*

I was half way through my lunch when the hostess arrived at my elbow again. 'I'm sorry, doctor, but the man with the sore neck is asking for you again. The Captain passes his respects and has asked me to assure you that Atlantic Airlines will suitably reimburse you for the inconvenience.' I sighed, standing again on the aisle man's toes. He glared at me. I followed her to the front of the huge airliner, *just a Greyhound bus with wings*, I thought, not guessing that this

93

small act of kindness would radically change my future holiday plans.

The captain was in the small cabin and, after shaking my hand, introduced me to the patient. 'This is Hubert J. Whyte Jr., doctor. I'm sure you have heard of him. He is the president of THC.' I should have been impressed but I had neither heard of Hubert J. Whyte Jr., nor the Tin Hat Corporation, but I nodded vaguely. The rich and famous take it amiss if you say you have never heard of them. He was just another patient with one of the most painful conditions that challenge Chiropractic physicians, as the American chiropractors like to be called. A patient who was disturbing my much needed holiday. I spoke to myself firmly: *Just get on with it, Bernie. Do your job. He needs your help.* The *real* doctor was nowhere in sight.

'Mr Whyte, would you please sit on this chair?' I carefully went through the active and passive ranges of motion of his neck again, did a few orthopaedic and neurological tests, motion palpation and a very quick myofascial examination. Although I didn't have the tools of my trade, the edge of the hand works reasonably well for a reflex hammer and a safety pin for a Wartenberg pinwheel. It didn't take long to establish that the Triceps muscle was already going weak, and I could see the *fasciculations** in the muscle; he jumped when I pricked parts of his arm, particularly the thumb and forefinger; the skin had become hypersensitive. I finished with a general palpation of the neck and armpit. The pulse in the Carotid artery was still regular and strong. This was no heart attack. Reminders from the past kept flashing through my mind, this time my Clinical Pathology lecturer of twenty-five years ago: *'If you don't look for it, the chances are good you won't find it.'* How right he was.

---

* Twitches in a muscle.

The examination had probably taken nearly ten minutes. All the while I was acutely conscious that my patient was in considerable pain, writhing and moving his arm and neck trying desperately to find a more comfortable position, despite the injection. In my experience only morphine drugs reduced the severe pain of a trapped nerve, and most relief – still only marginal – was found by placing the arm over the head. The patient was a good looking man in his early forties and for the first time I noted the cut of his clothes, the complete absence of designer labels, the heavy gold chain and a general air of affluence.

'Mr Whyte, the pain in your arm is coming from a pinched nerve here in your neck.' I prodded using the *touch and tell* technique that we chiropractors love. 'It is affecting your arm as you can feel. It is a very painful and serious condition, most likely caused by the way you were sleeping on the flight over from Johannesburg.

'The airline seat! You mean the seat was the cause of all this pain?' Mr Whyte said. The Captain moved uneasily. I wondered why he was still there, almost guarding his passenger, my patient.

'Oh, there's almost certainly old injury in your neck, but your sleeping posture was most likely the cause of this episode.'

'Yes, I had an automobile accident about ten years ago. It didn't cause much pain at the time. Within a week or two the pain in my neck had gone.' He looked at me questioningly, tilting his head upwards and flinching at the sharp jab of pain in his arm.

'Were you examined by a chiropractor?' Silently I laughed at myself. *Just trying to get more mileage out of the injury, Bernie. Remember you are on holiday. You will never see this man again.* I was wrong.

'No, I just went to the emergency room. They said it was a mild whiplash and would get better of its own accord. It did,' he finished indignantly.

'It's one of the mysteries of whiplash,' I said. 'The pain usually goes away after a few days or a week, but the subluxation, or fixation as we sometimes call it, that is caused by the accident remains and then degenerative change sets in. This is frequently the result. It's not yet proven but we believe that if you had it treated at the time that this would have been much less likely to occur.'

'Hmff,' he expostulated, thinking about what I had said.

'You mean every person should be examined by a chiropractor after a whiplash?' It was the first time the captain had contributed anything since introducing me to Mr Whyte.

'We think so, but then we are biased!' I laughed. 'I'm not licensed in America so I can't treat you, Mr Whyte,' I said, turning back to my patient. He was rubbing his arm trying to get some relief, before placing it above his head again. 'But I will do some gentle traction and mobilization of your neck, and cross friction of these muscles in spasm.' I palpated the Scalenii muscles in his neck, and he winced.

'What do you mean you can't treat me? It's my neck that's at risk, isn't it?'

'Yes, it is but it still wouldn't be wise,' I said thinking of my own neck. 'This is a serious condition and is not likely to resolve for some weeks, even a few months for the strength to return to your arm. I would insist on an x-ray in my practice and an MRI if you had the money.'

'The money!' he said scornfully. 'Do you know who I am?'

'No sir, I don't, but it makes no difference who you are. I am, in effect, an unlicensed chiropractor and you have a serious problem. We'll be in New York in... I turned to the Captain... in how many hours?'

'Now just you listen to me, doctor. I just want you to click my neck. Now! I can't stand this pain any longer.'

I pondered that for a moment. The man was obviously used to getting his way when he shouted 'jump'. 'How long Captain?'

The Captain looked uncertainly at his watch. 'A little over three hours.'

'You mean I have to endure this pain for another three hours just because this man doesn't have the balls to treat me!' I winced at that but he was speaking to the Captain, and then turned to me. 'You're just like the rest of the stupid medics. Terrified of being sued. Call yourself a doctor!'

For just a moment I thought of a Canadian woman I had been treating recently. I am not known for being a heavy-handed chiropractor, but she had said: 'I have been to at least six chiropractors in Canada and the U.S. and none of them were as vigorous as you! Four of them wouldn't even adjust my neck like you do.' Could it be that, because of the threat of being sued, chiropractors in the Americas have become so gentle, lacking the courage to intervene in the forceful way needed to address a serious spinal injury? Men without balls? Or was he just being manipulative? One thing I knew for certain was that the sooner a serious condition was treated the more likely there was going to be a beneficial outcome.

The Captain intervened again. 'Doctor, if you were in a remote part of South Africa where you are licensed, but where no x-rays were readily available, would you adjust a patient with this condition?'

I considered that one. It was an unexpected turn. 'Yes, I probably would. It increases the risk not having a clear picture but, yes, I probably would.'

'Then get on and do it,' growled Hubert J. Whyte Jr. 'Damn it all, I'll sign a Good Samaritan affidavit freeing you of responsibility.'

I knew I was being bullied by a man who was used to people complying when he commanded but agreed that it was a reasonable request. It was a fateful moment, one that in fact was to make me famous, but not until after a vast amount of work. It didn't stop me covering my butt, though. There was no guarantee he would be any better after one adjustment, or in a happier frame of mind, and in fact sometimes the condition would get worse before it resolved. 'Captain, would you find out if there is an attorney on board who would put together a simple affidavit freeing me from all responsibility, and stating there would be no charge for the service. Meantime I'll go and wash up and get some oil.' I knew that I had a small vial of Arnica in my hand luggage.

I had treated several hundreds of cases of serious Brachial Neuralgias over the years, perhaps even thousands, so I was able to move confidently and efficiently. Despite not having x-rays, I knew that mostly they showed disc degeneration in the lower cervical spine, probably between C5 and 6, possibly an old compression fracture, and most likely encroachment into the *foramen* from which the nerve emerges. The numbness in his thumb and forefinger told me exactly where the problem was. Though never a routine condition, I was confident in my ability. The possibility of cancer of the spine, infection or an extra-dural tumour was remote. The condition presented in the exact classical way.

'Miracles we do at once, the impossible takes a little longer,' my partner used to say to patients who expected instant relief. I said my prayers but was still astonished to hear later how quickly Hubert J. Whyte Jr. responded to just one Chiropractic adjustment.

I was quite tense when we landed, and appreciated the way Atlantic Airlines management whisked me through the formalities. Cousin $ue was there to meet me. I was looking forward to the long drive to New Hampshire. It was many years since my favourite cousin and I had been able to spend ten hours of quality time together. Why did she spell her name with a $? Probably like all of us hoping that a few millions of the lolly by that name would end up in her account. Unfortunately that would never happen to me with only one pair of hands, nor her as a scientist. The world never rewarded people like us in that way. Hubert J. Whyte Jr. did help indirectly though: American Airlines did finally accede to my request to do some research into neck and back pain after overnight flights.

Chapter Ten

IT'S NOT WHAT YOU KNOW THAT COUNTS.

There is a healthy way to be ill.

Dr George Sheehan

My father had aged in the ten years since I had last seen him. So had I, I reminded myself. Nevertheless I was shocked. Thirty years of abusive drinking and twenty-plus cigarettes a day had taken its toll. Actually it was a miracle he was still alive; a miracle due in part to the fact that he ate so well and walked at least five kilometres every day, whatever the weather. It was Alcoholics Anonymous, though, that had saved his life but too late to save his marriage to my mother. She never married again; and neither did he. It was my father who had taught me the value of fruit for breakfast and a chopped green salad every day, preferably with assorted yellows, reds, purples and any other colours where the beta-carotenes are found. Now in his old age he spent every day in the summer digging and potting in his veggie garden. During the long American winters Pops grew Mung bean sprouts and the like, and ate the dozens of jars of canned apples, green beans and pickled beets that he had grown and put up; there were never any white elephants under the Christmas tree from the family patriarch. That was provided for, in the main, by his organic garden, from which they could never get enough, and the family obviously loved him.

It was good to see my father again and we hugged one another with much back-slapping and the loud shouts and cheers that the Americans so love. My mother was very

English and I never entirely lost her more thoughtful and reserved nature. Dad was a man's man and I loved him despite his weaknesses, even the one I had inherited. I had a stack of handwritten letters, sent faithfully every week that kept us nearly as close as if he lived next door. Dad's philosophy was that parents may divorce their spouses, but never their children. After one particularly brutal drunken beating, my mother had left him, returning with Alan and me to her native South Africa where we built new lives. Alan moved back to the States after finishing his schooling.

Later, after I had unpacked and taken a much needed shower, we sat down for a traditional American supper. Just as we were finishing the apple pie, before the coffee was served, the phone rang shrilly, disturbing the rowdy dinner. Dad handed me the phone: 'It's for you, Bernie.'

I wondered who knew I was here, in far off Charter's Creek. Helen, certainly, but who else? 'Ah, Mr Whyte. How are you?' I winked to the dozen or so relatives sitting around the old Walnut table. I wondered: *How did he get my number?*

'Much better, eh. That's good. I still recommend you see a chiropractor tomorrow. Rome wasn't built in a day you know.' I smiled at the crew. They were all watching and listening. I was surprised how one phone call could stop a bunch of noisy Americans in their tracks.

'Anything you can do? No, of course not, I was just happy to be of help.' I nodded to the family while Hubert J. Whyte Jr. continued.

'Well, that's very kind of you, Mr Whyte but I'm afraid I won't be here long enough to take you up on Colorado. Perhaps a rain cheque? I'm an abominable skier anyway. I would probably break *my* neck!' I grinned and they could all hear Hubert J. Whyte laughing at the other end of the phone.

'Mr Whyte, actually there is something you might be able to do. I don't know how much weight you carry but I was hoping Atlantic Airlines might consider allowing me to do some research on neck pain during and after overnight flights. If I were to contact you, would you give me your support? ...You would? Well, that's very gracious of you. Have you got an email address?' More smiles around the table; they were still all ears.

'You mean you're in *Who's Who* in America? Gee, you must be a man of some influence, Mr Whyte. That's very good of you. When I have put together a proposal to the Airline, I'll be in contact. Meantime, perhaps you could make a discreet call or two? Thank you very much. Goodbye, Mr Whyte.'

'Who was that, Bernie?' Dad asked, seemingly casual.

'Oh, just some guy I helped on the plane. He had a sore neck.'

'Some guy?' asked $ue. 'It's not every man that's in *Who's Who*.'

'Wasn't Hubert J. Whyte, Jr. by any chance, was it Bernie?' asked Dad quietly.

'How did you know that, Pops?' I asked, using my childhood name for him.

$ue interrupted: 'He's one of the ten richest men in America, Bernie! Do you mean you treated Hubert J. Whyte, Jr. on the plane? He's in the same league as the Rockefellers and Bill Gates.'

I went white. Cold too, a little frisson of astonishment travelling the length of my spine. 'You must be joking? One of the richest men in America! I wondered why the Captain stayed with us the whole time I was examining and treating him. Omigosh!'

The family talk went on into the late hours. They wanted to know about Helen and why she hadn't come. 'Just couldn't afford it, this time, I'm afraid, folks. Not after we had paid for the kids at private schools.'

'Couldn't afford it! Why didn't you say so? And what's the matter with your practice anyway? Chiropractors are mostly rich people here.' The wine was loosening $ue's inhibitions and she spoke her mind rather too readily.

'I'm afraid I only charge the equivalent of $10 per consultation and, with our high rate of tax, anything that's priced in dollars – like airline flights – is very expensive.'

'Then why do you live there? Why don't you also come back to the States?' asked my brother Alan.

'Because we have the best soaring in the world,' I replied, putting my tongue out at him just like we did when we were kids. We all laughed and the conversation moved on to American, Middle Eastern and finally Zimbabwean politics. Alan and his wife Shelley had joined Helen and me at a glorious Victoria Falls holiday some ten years previously.

'I saw a black lady saying on TV: "Life was profoundly better under Ian Smith than under Robert Mugabe." Is that true?'

'Without a doubt unless you are one of Mugabe's aides but let's stay away from politics. I don't trust many politicians, black or white. They're mostly a self-serving lot with their own personal agendas. Do you trust your own President?' There was a palpable silence around the table as they rolled their eyes and scowled but nobody said a word. I knew they were mainly Republicans.

'Enough of this for the old men. I'm off to bed. I'll see you all in the morning,' said Dad. 'Bernie, grab a coffee and come and tuck me in like I used to do for you.' He gave me a wink. How I loved the man despite the hardship his drinking had brought to my childhood.

Americans know how to make coffee and I took a mug from the ever-ready pot. Fortunately coffee doesn't keep me awake. My bed too was calling so I said my good nights to the family, thinking how like my Tammy, Alan's Jenny looked. They would have been friends, if fate hadn't placed an ocean between them. They might be one day yet. $ue and my English cousin George were counted amongst my best friends. I wound my way up the carpeted stairs to Dad's bedroom on the second floor and sat in a comfortable rocking chair looking out over the lake, sipping the hot liquid while he did his ablutions. I remembered being rocked in the same chair nearly fifty years ago, hidden in my father's dressing gown. Moonlight was twinkling off a thousand mirrors on the water at the far side of the cove. It was good to be home, only it wasn't home any longer. It was my father who had taught me that home is where you hang up your hat, and that was in far off Africa, not New Hampshire.

'Son, I have to make an important decision in the next week or two.'

I swivelled around in my chair, facing him. He was tucked up in bed with the spot-light above his head shining down onto where he would normally be reading. I approved. It was where I had told him to fit it. Bedside lights may be very chic but they are definitely not made for reading. The lamp was not too high so he could easily reach the switch and not too low where he might scratch his head. He had told me in various emails about the neck pain that wasn't responding to Chiropractic treatment, and I had suggested he think about posture, starting with his pillows and sleeping position. I waited, recognizng that it was something important.

'I have an aneurysm. A big one.' He pointed to the lower abdominal region. 'My doctor says I should have it operated on.'

I felt the second cold shudder of the evening. 'How big, Pops?'

'I don't know but they tell me it could burst at any time. The scans are over there on the table.'

I got up and, picking up the envelope, pulled out the report. There was plenty of time to look at the scans themselves tomorrow. 'Seven centimetres, Pops. Big, but not huge.' A sudden weariness came over me. I looked at my watch. 'It's 7am on my time-clock, Pops. Let me sleep on it and we'll talk tomorrow.'

We sat in a comfortable silence. He was the first to break it: 'You're looking tired, Bernie. Is everything okay?'

I nodded. 'I work too hard and running a solo practice all those years was plain stupid. I could never take a proper holiday.'

'And now how is the new practice doing?'

'As you know, I'm sure I told you in one of my letters, I joined practices with an elderly chiropractor who also wanted more time for herself. Then we hired a young gun and things are much better.'

'Still work too hard, though?'

I nodded. 'But at least now I can take longer holidays. Like this one,' I added.

We sat quietly for another few minutes, I thinking of the time-bomb ticking away in my father's abdomen. He was thinking about my practice: 'Has it created tensions forming this super-practice?'

I pondered that: 'Yes, it has but she was absolutely insistent that we draw up a water-tight contract. She was once ripped off by a young buck that she hired and didn't want to make the same mistake. He did his damnedest to hijack her practice. Once bitten, twice shy and all that, but now everything is exactly proscribed in the contract. When we will appear for work, how much leave we can take, how the bonus system works. Everything. Actually, it has made life much easier and our new associate, Scott, has his heart in the right place.' I yawned.

'It's past your bedtime.' We both laughed; I still remember those self same words from the days of my childhood. 'Before you go, is all well with Helen and my grandchildren? It's time they met their grandfather, you know. I'm not going to live forever,' he finished, meaningfully.

I walked over and sat on the edge of his bed. 'They're fine. I'll tell you all about them tomorrow.' We looked at each other for long moments and I felt hot tears forming in the corners of my eyes. I reached out and hugged him, before silently leaving his bedroom not trusting myself to speak again.

It was a long night: jetlag, the exhaustion of too many demanding months at the clinic and the stress of Hubert J Whyte Jr and his painful neck all conspired to disrupt my circadian rhythms. Meeting my family again after so many years, too much beer and coffee and now the shock of my father's aneurysm, also took their toll. Despite the normal environmental cues my time-clocks were chiming 'it's wake up time'. It is not surprising that jetlag is known to throw susceptible people into a severe depression. Finally I fell into a fitful sleep but nightmares of Christo, one of my favourite

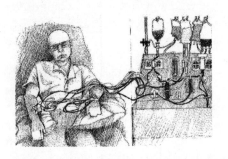

patients, kept waking me in a sweat. First Dad had Christo's face and was lying in a hospital ward, an oxygen mask over his face and with various tubes and monitor cables running to and from his body. Then Christo was gardening in Dad's patch. It was a disturbed and disturbing night, not nearly long enough, but then also far too long. I couldn't wait for morning.

Most patients you like. Some you can't help disliking. A few you could love. Christo I admired. Actually, I liked him a lot, one of those clean, upright elderly men whom everybody respected. Christo suffered from an embarrassing condition called Alopecia Areata, that caused large patches of his hair to fall out. Eventually he just shaved his head. I knew he wasn't on any fad diets, known to cause Alopecia, but his doctor and I had to consider some other diseases like Diabetes, Lupus and Thyroid conditions, none of which he had. We eventually agreed that it was probably a side-effect of his blood pressure medication that, along with many other drugs, was known to cause Alopecia occasionally.

My training had tried to teach me to remain slightly aloof, separate from, distant perhaps from my patients. But Christo was a man I had grown to respect deeply and remaining aloof had proved impossible. He had first been referred to me by my young associate, Scott.

Most patients respond to Chiropractic treatment whether you feel a click or not. My theory is that usually both the doctor and the patient feel or hear the *release*, as we call it. Occasionally only the doctor or only the patient feels it, the sound muffled perhaps by *adipose* tissue. Sometimes neither the patient nor the doctor feels the release, but motion palpation after the adjustment confirms whether the joint has, in fact, moved. But Christo hadn't been getting better with Scott's treatment and neither he nor Christo had been hearing releases.

Christo was an elderly man who had retired early from the public service. Basically he was retrenched because he was white in a South Africa now intent on levelling the playing fields. Making reparations for an ugly Apartheid past that prevented black South Africans from getting promotion, even if they were able, was only fair – unless it went on indefinitely. Christo was one of those who paid the price for two generations of racial wickedness. He wasn't bitter, knowing that he had benefited from Apartheid and, in any case, he was loving his early retirement.

He had taken a bad fall outside his kitchen door one day when the steps were slippery and injured his spine. For some reason I was able to adjust him, where Scott had failed, and Christo responded well. He was pain free within six weeks of treatment and eternally grateful.

He was a wonderfully healthy and active man. He was able to play golf twice a week again, he went salmon fishing on the South Coast at least once a month and, he and his wife, went caravanning to the Cape to visit their daughter for two months every year. The trip always started with a drive through the Northern Cape to enjoy the spectacular Namaqualand daisies in the Spring, followed by a quiet tow down through the Boland to their daughter's wine farm at Franschhoek. He had one skeleton in his cupboard: Christo had been a smoker for fifty years. Under my bullying he had stopped, but all the years on the weed had left its mark on his blood vessels.

'Christo, it's been five years since you were x-rayed and it's time for a new series. In any case, as you know, your back has not been behaving as well recently. Please have these films taken in the next week or two. There's no urgency.' I handed Christo the requisition and he did not demur. I had won his respect and he did what I asked without hesitation, despite the cost. Christo would have to dig into his pension.

A few weeks later, as I opened the packet of x-rays, neither Christo nor I anticipated the finding. I spent long minutes looking first at the plates and then reading the report, twice. 'Christo, I'm afraid this is not good news. You have a large aneurysm in the artery that supplies your legs and your lower abdomen. They have recommended you have an ultrasound scan so we can determine exactly how large the aneurysm is. It's the right decision.'

Healthy, strong, life-loving Christo died of complications three weeks after the surgery. First he went into kidney failure and then a clot to the lung finished him. I never forgave myself for recommending he go for the operation. Nor did his wife forgive me: her instincts had been right, but Christo followed the advice of his doctors and his chiropractor.

I tossed and turned all night. By 6am my clocks were telling me it was mid afternoon and that bed was not the place to be. I got up quietly and slipped downstairs taking my Bible and journal that went everywhere with me, even round the world. I had to hunt for tea in the solid oak kitchen. Americans don't drink much tea, and even then it's usually iced in the summer. I paged back to the days of Christo's death and re-read my entry: *'Think twice, no six times, before sending an elderly person for major, and even minor, surgery.'*

The days passed in a blur. Dad and I did not discuss his aneurysm again until the morning before I left. I was avoiding the subject, as did the rest of the family, and I despised myself for it. My father needed some straight forward advice: the loneliness of the sick, nobody wants to talk about their illnesses, not even his son who was in the business of health.

'You've been avoiding the subject of my aneurysm, Bernie, haven't you? You've got to help me, my boy.' We were sitting in his bedroom again. I stared out over the cove again, trying to evade his direct question.

'I'm damned if I do and damned if I don't, Pops,' I admitted.

'What do you mean?'

'Well, there's no right and wrong answer. Only what's right for you.'

'Explain.'

I took a deep breath and tried to marshal my thoughts. It wasn't easy. 'Let's start from the standpoint that either way you are going to die, Pops. Sooner or later.' He winced at that. I marvelled at the sheer power of the elderly to cling to life. Life was obviously good and he was not ready to face death, but yes, Pops was going to die. I wasn't ready to face his death either. 'So am I,' I said looking him in the eye, smiling, 'perhaps even before you, if I carry on with the life of the mad creature that I am.'

'Yes, that may be true,' he said in his American drawl, finally exclaiming: 'but it doesn't help me any!'

For a moment I wondered what had happened to my childhood accent. Finally after five years in Africa I had stopped saying to'ma-to and had started saying to-maat'-o. 'I'm afraid the blunt answer is simply this: It's a dangerous and risky procedure, Pops. The anaesthetic could knock out a few million marbles and there's a fair chance you may die on the table. My advice, Pops, is to avoid the operation and to prepare yourself for sudden death. It's going to happen sooner or later. In every other respect you are a very healthy seventy-year-old. Keep your blood pressure under control and there's a reasonable chance the artery won't pop for five or more years, or you'll die of something else.

Jenny, my niece, knocked on the door. 'I'm not horning in on anything, am I?' she asked with a smile. She was drinking plain bottled water rather than our coffee. I admired the new generation – there's nothing wrong with drinking water. Why should it always be tea or coffee or cola?

'No, you're certainly not and maybe you can contribute another viewpoint. Your grandfather has a seven centimetre aortic aneurysm and he's asked my opinion.' Jenny was in fifth-year medicine.

I went on to tell them about Christo and the guilt I felt, having sent him to his death. 'The surgeon will probably tell you that I am being highly irresponsible for suggesting to you that you don't have the operation. The doctor's side of the picture is that tomorrow could be a *sudden death* day, or even today, and it's not got anything to do with golf.' I grinned at Dad. He had thrashed me on the golf course a few days after I arrived. 'The surgeon could be right, maybe I am. What do you think, Jenny?'

She didn't answer for a while. She knew about the aneurysm, my father wasn't the kind to be secretive about such things, but it was the first time she had really faced that her grandfather was going to die, maybe quite soon. I could see from the way she looked at him, the way she had cuddled with him over the last three weeks, that he wasn't only my favourite. He was one of those men adored by his whole family since he had joined Alcoholics Anonymous and completely given up all booze. Finally she contributed: 'Do you think a regular ultra-sound scan, taken every few months, would warn us if the aneurism was expanding?'

'Excellent, Jen!' I said. 'Excellent idea.' I was not a little irritated with myself for not thinking of it first. It was after all obvious. 'Smart granddaughter you have there, Pops,' I said to him with a wink.

Jenny ignored me. 'I'll do a search of the internet for some statistics and, when I get back to med school, I'll talk to the profs. What are the chances of a seventy-year-old man with controlled blood pressure, still smoking' – she scowled at him for a moment, before grinning again – 'dying from a burst seven-centimetre abdominal aneurysm in the next five years?'

'And, statistically what are the chances of me surviving the operation, but with the sudden onset of senile dementia?' my father asked worriedly.

My father never had that operation. He dropped dead in his garden, some seven years later, trowel in hand with his faithful Wire-haired Terrier at his feet. It was she who summoned my brother Alan. I envied Dad that death, quick and clean – it beat, hands down the sterile, but desperately lonely, white-washed ward of the best hospital where so many of us are doomed to die. He was well prepared for the long-expected day, having no need to *shed bitter tears over graves for words left unsaid or deeds left undone.*[*] Only my mother still harboured angry feelings towards him, and that not surprisingly. It was more than two years before I saw my father again, though we continued to correspond regularly, and call occasionally. He enjoyed more years than I expected. For once Bernard Preston got it right.

---

[*] Harriet Beecher Stowe, abolitionist and novelist (1811–1896)

During the whole three weeks in New Hampshire the family plagued me. Fortunately, I love my work, but on holiday it was indeed something of a labour of love. 'Bernie, do you think you could look at my back? It hurts.' That was Alan's son – he had a dreadful scoliosis. 'Bernie, can Chiropractic help headaches?' My sister-in-law spent at least one day a week holed up in a dark room and two more days suffering. I was shocked at how many analgesics she was taking. Dad had thoracic pain from so much coughing, Jenny too was suffering from headaches. Colin had pain in the ankle that was threatening his athletic career. The whole family seemed to have need for Chiropractic treatment for one ailment or another. They queued up every day, only one member of the family, $ue, consulting a chiropractor with any regularity. Why, in the land of *Daniel D. Palmer*[*], a land with nearly 70,000 chiropractors, their own relative in the business, were they not consulting their local chiropractor? They wouldn't talk about it and it was only some months later that I discovered quite by accident the reason why.

---

[*] Founder of Chiropractic in 1895.

Chapter Eleven

ISITHU-THUTHU

If a man happens to find himself, he has a mansion which he can inhabit with dignity all the days of his life.

James Michener

I've always been an early bird. Even before the effects of jetlag had worn off I was still the first awake and out of bed in my American home by at least an hour. Jenny was usually the first to disturb the peace of what I call *Selfish Hour*[*] and it was often another half hour before anyone else appeared. Jenny was also a Christian, the only other believer in my pagan American family.

'Have you seen this?' she asked me one morning. She lugged out a huge tome that could only be laid flat inside the old oak bookcase that my grandfather had once made for his bride far back in the last millennium. Being interested in carpentry myself, I had admired the old piece, which was beautifully crafted with an intricate leaded stained-glass pattern on the doors, but I had missed the book. I did wonder how Granddad had worked the edges of the cabinet without all the modern tools that I used in my workshop. The book was an ancient family Bible. We pored over it together, looking at the names of the Preston clan going back nearly two hundred years. It was an eerie feeling tracing the names of these forgotten forebears whose genes we still bore. The book was written in quaint old English but I recognized the stark power of the words where I had randomly opened the

---

[*] Reference: *Frog in my Throat.*

113

old book: *'Behold, I stand at the door and knock: if any man hear my voice...'*[*]

That too had an eerie feeling. I had unerringly opened the old book at the words that had brought me to Christ so many years ago. Quietly I thanked Him for the courage given to *open that door;* it had been both stubbornly difficult, the door handle found only on the inside, my side, and yet also remarkably easy. Best of all was the many times we had *supped* together. *Are you saying something, Lord?* Why had Jenny brought me the old book? As I thumbed through its pages it suddenly dawned on me: 'You know what, Jenny? This book has never been read.' The pages were crisp and clean despite being nearly two centuries old. No one in the Preston clan had ever delved into the life-giving pages! For a moment I reflected on one of my common clinic sayings to patients: 'These back exercises are a bit like a Bible – quite useless if stuck in the bookcase, but life and health-giving when used regularly.'

Pops' birthday party was a grand affair. Alan had decided that Patrick's Place was just right. In the proper Irish tradition it was decorated in green and gold but with the boating and fishing themes strong; life-buoys and lobster pots. Fishnets adorned the walls along with small prints of New England seabirds. Pride of place was a mural of an Irish-looking mermaid with wild, dark hair and good looks, her scales made from shells found on the New England seashore. Pitchers of strong American beer, accompanied by platters of lobster tails and even unexpected Alaskan Crab legs, together with bottles of Californian white wines got the party moving. The succulent flesh, pried out with crackers and forks and dipped in hot melted butter had my mouth watering for more. Course after course of traditional American fare: Seafood Gumbo and hot bread rolls, fresh from the oven, pork and beans with apple sauce and Boston

---

[*] The Bible, Revelations chapter 3

butt; piles of fresh salads and coleslaw, apple pie and cheesecake and hot filter-coffee to finish it off. I noticed, not a little guiltily, that my father didn't touch the alcohol.

The American champagne was not up to our JC le Roux but by then not many of us noticed. The toasts to my father's long life brought out the gifts from a family who obviously adored their patriarch. A pure lamb's wool sweater from Scotland and an Irish tam-o'-shanter, a new set of stainless steel gardening tools and a galvanised watering can, several books including one of my favourites: *Kitchen Table Wisdom* and, of course, the inevitable CDs from the grandchildren.

'Pops, my gift to you is something that is already yours. It is your birthright but you've never appropriated it!' I pulled out the old tome that I had brought with me to the restaurant. 'It was first purchased by your great grandfather John Preston in 1803 when he married Pretty Maggie Thomas,' I read out the details. 'All the names of our forebears are written here on the fly-cover as you know – I'm sure you've read them many times. But the best part of this book is not its antiquity, nor the history of our family, but the life that Jesus gives to those who read it. It's my gift to you along with this bookmark of your African family.' Everyone looked a bit embarrassed except Pops who looked me straight in the eye: 'Thank you, Bernie. I'll start reading it tonight,' he said taking the old family Bible, handling it for just a moment with his rough gardener's hands before adding it to the growing pile at his elbow.

It wasn't long before the general hubbub, which had started up again, was drowned out by a dozen or so sleek and shiny Harleys rumbling in. I looked at them longingly, wishing I could at least take one around the parking lot, but I knew that bikes are like toothbrushes: you don't lend them to anyone. Not *anyone* and certainly not to this unlicensed foreigner. The low throaty roars of the bikes got my juices going, like the smell of hot fresh bread. Alan hailed one of the riders, obviously one of his pals, in a heavy black leather jacket and a colourful blue bandanna dotted with yellow stars around his head. Americans love their stars. 'Hey, Tom, come and meet my family.' The huge bear of a man came across and congratulated Pops on his day and then worked his way around the group. I was last.

'Hi, Tom, it's good to meet you. Would you take me for a short spin around the block before you leave?'

Tom looked at me keenly: 'You a biker?'

'How did you know?' I laughed. 'Is it that obvious?'

'Yeah, it is,' he said, in a voice that sounded not unlike the burbling rumble that his bike made. 'Whataya ride?' this in the vernacular.

'I've got an ancient BMW, though I call her *isithuthuthu*,' I replied in mine. 'The thousand.'

He smiled as I said it, the lovely syllables with all the clicks rolling off my tongue. 'What on earth does that mean?'

I grinned back. Having learnt Zulu as a child I could enunciate the difficult sounds correctly. 'Simply a motor cycle. Nice, eh?'

More soberly he asked: 'The tourer?'

'No, mine's got the small fairing. My *dream machine*.'

He nodded. 'I know the bike. We only ride Harleys here.'

He looked at me for a long moment: ''Fraid I can't take you out today, but I tell you what. How about joining us tomorrow for a ride up to Mount Washington?'

'You serious? I'd absolutely love to.'

'You're on,' he said. 'Tracey's got her own bike,' he said, gesturing at his wife sitting with their friends, 'so you can ride pillion behind me.' We made a few arrangements of place and time and Tom said his farewells and went back to his friends.

'Gee, Alan, you've really made my day by introducing me to Tom.'

'No better way to see the New Hampshire,' he said, 'but I'd better find you a warm jacket.' The fall chill was setting in and I looked forward to seeing the New England colours.

It was a memorable day, not just because it was my first ride on a Harley. Nor because of lunch at the famous Mount Washington Hotel or the ride up the mountain in the tooth-wheeled train. Mostly it was memorable because of the ride home. We were speeding down a long straight and, as we leaned into the bend, Tom's wife, Tracey, riding a *Fat Boy** hit a slick of diesel and wrapped her leg around a maple tree. Tom and I were first there. Tracey was groaning in agony, holding her lower leg which was obviously broken. 'Get onto your cell, Tom. Get an ambulance.'

I carefully loosened Tracey's trousers and Tom wanted to start cutting a slit in her leggings with a fierce looking flick-knife. 'Don't Tom. Her pants will keep it clean.' The skin was clearly broken and the blood was already soaking through her trouser leg. Fortunately, one of the group had a first aid box, so I quickly applied an inadequate dressing, tightening her trouser leg again and Tom applied pressure with a spare T-shirt to stem the bleeding. It was a compound fracture of both the tibia and fibula, mid-shaft so, while I gently stabilised her leg, one of the others with some first aid experience found a small roll-up mattress that had been brought for the trip. We loosely applied it to Tracey's leg, giving support. She was beginning to go into shock, both deathly pale and sweating profusely but she was quite lucid, asking questions about the injury. I instructed them to use their jackets to keep her warm. Fortunately the pulses in the leg were normal so we just made her as comfortable as we could. 'Any other big pains, Tracey?'

'Yes, my shoulder's a bit sore and this knee is the devil.' She pointed to her knee just above the fracture site. I was tempted to test the ligaments, knowing from my medico-legal work that the soft tissues are often neglected in South African trauma centres, especially when there has been bony fracture but decided against it. Bones heal but ruptured ligaments, if

---

* Popular model of Harley-Davidson motorcycle.

not attended to, will leave the patient with a weak and disabled joint for life. The knee too was already beginning to swell alarmingly. She had a few tender spots around her shoulder but nothing else obviously wrong. A complete examination later was obviously imperative: an undetected ruptured spleen could prove fatal.

'Tom, make sure the orthopod deals with her knee as well as the fractures,' I said. 'By the look of how quickly that knee is swelling, she could have an injury to a cruciate ligament. If it isn't treated she will end up with a very unstable knee.'

The whites of his eyes revealed his fear. 'What's going to happen to Tracey? Is she going to be okay?'

'They will probably put a nail down the centre of her leg – at least that's how a tibial fracture is treated in South Africa,' I said. 'It's messy but quite routine. Occasionally it might need a plate. But the ligaments in her knee are a lot more complicated. She'll probably be in hospital for a week or two and then on crutches for about two months, maybe longer. For heaven's sake, don't let her walk on the leg until the surgeon says it's okay, otherwise the nail can slip up into the knee.'

Just then we heard the sound of sirens and it wasn't long before the paramedics had Tracey in the ambulance on a drip. They roared off into the early evening traffic. Twelve motorcycles and eleven licensed riders were left at the scene. And me. Several of Tom's pals had been checking out Tracey's machine: it had a few scratches but otherwise it was fine. Tom looked at me: 'Looks like you're going to get that ride, Bernie. We'll ride in a bunch and you just stay in the centre. And remember to stay on the right-hand side of the road,' he finished with a chuckle.

We arrived back in Charter's Creek long after dark. The accident had a sobering effect on the gang and everyone rode very sedately home. It was a serious breach of the American law but I had driven a car on the right hand side of the road for more than three years in Chicago, and I had at least 100,000 kilometres credit on my BMW dream machine. The ride was uneventful and I loved every minute. Tom's Harley handled beautifully and the throbbing burble from the twin exhausts had me exhilarated. Tracey's leg was well managed by the surgeon and within six months was almost normal. It could have been a lot worse, and I got my ride on a big fast *Hawg.*[*]

My last few days in America arrived. We were having a breakfast of flap-jacks and maple syrup, with large dollops of cream, followed by ham and eggs. Eggs with an 's' – everybody in America has to have at least two. There was a hoot from outside and Alan went to see, coming back with an envelope for me from a courier.

I opened it. Slowly my mouth opened wide, my eyes too, they told me later. 'Well, what is it?' asked Alan.

I passed it to Pops. He reached for his glasses and the smile spread across his face too. 'An open Atlantic Airlines return ticket for two from Johannesburg to Denver, and a week in the Marriott penthouse at Vail, courtesy of Hubert J. Whyte, Jr. and Atlantic Airlines.' The whole family cheered and Jenny shouted: 'I'm going to send an email to Helen. Now I'll get to meet her.'

---

[*] American name/slang for a big fast Harley-Davidson.

Chapter Twelve

I'M INTO LUMBAR, TOO.

*The only problem with progress
is that it goes forwards instead of backwards.*

Oscar Wilde

Alan had heard that the early Prestons came from the Cape Cod area, where the first Pilgrims landed in America, so we decided to spend my last two days grave-digging. Armed with as much information as we could get hold of, we set off just after dawn, armed with a Thermos of strong brewed coffee and a cardboard box of nasty donuts that the Americans do so love. The road took us towards Boston and then south to the Cape, where we crossed over a wide canal; it cut an ugly swathe through the natural beauty of the sandy peninsula that reached out into the Atlantic like a giant crooked arm, reminding us of the so-called progress that can sometimes be obscene.

We drove through forests and between the rough dunes and marshes that separated the little villages. Everywhere there were signs of a vibrant fishing industry and I couldn't wait to tuck into some oysters and scallops or perhaps a clam chowder, at lunch. Graveyards have never been my forte but, once we started discovering the early Prestons, connecting this part of the family with that, and finally the first George and his wife, Pretty Martha's, grave, we started whooping around like two kids who had just found the Easter Bunny. Our excursion ended in Plymouth's Mayflower Society Museum. Our family was full of Georges and Johns and their Pretty wives.

'Well actually, I'm afraid that George Preston was the ship's doctor on *The Anne* which arrived ten years after the *Mayflower*. You are certainly descents of the early settlers, but you are not eligible to become members of the Mayflower Society,' the researcher smiled at us. No doubt she had dealt with thousands of hopefuls so the hangdog look on our faces didn't surprise her.

We wandered around the garden and the period house next to the museum. I took a few measurements and made a sketch of a rocking chair I wanted to copy and Alan looked at old paintings of Tall Ships. He was the sailor in the family. We came to an oil of the master of the house and his wife.

'Do you think they really wore those clothes?' I asked. 'To breakfast?'

'Bet it was only when they were on show,' laughed Alan. He knew how hot and humid the New England summers could be. 'Beautiful lady though, nice figure,' he finished.

'Lady, ladies? Were there women on the *Mayflower*, Alan?'

'Of course, there were. No women, no descendents, clot.' He punched me lightly on the shoulder, just like old times.

'You don't get it, twit, do you? Is the museum still open?' The guide nodded looking at his watch. I pounded down the stairs with a bewildered Alan behind me and a very puzzled guide left at the top of the stairs, mid-sentence, about to describe the period four-poster bed.

'What on earth is this about, Bernie?'

'Just think, won't you! Could Pretty Martha or her parents could have been on the *Mayflower*?' Alan's eyes widened and he gasped: 'Why didn't we think of it?'

'One of us just did!' I retorted.

The rest is history. Pretty Martha's mother *was* on the *Mayflower*. She was the blacksmith's wife. We were true Mayflower descendants, but Alan had lots of paperwork to do to prove it. I had only one task: 'When you get to England, Bernie, see if you can get to the churchyard at

Brenchley's Green in Kent. George's father, Ebenezer, is buried there.' George was one of the *Ten Men of Kent*.[*]

Farewells are never easy, particularly when you know there is a good chance you may never see your father again. A hug, a sob and a dash for the car. 'Let's go, Alan.' Pops never did have his operation and died seven years later of a cerebral aneurysm in his garden, tending his blessed beets. He had a cigarette in his hand when he fell but I couldn't be angry with him. He had lived a long and full life, and was, in the end much loved and respected by family and friends. But his father died at eighty-seven, also from a stroke. Dad was lucky – it was quick and clean compared to the death that many smokers can expect but the weed had still robbed him of ten years of his life.

Large aeroplanes are a very boring mode of transport, but it's still the simplest way to get from Boston to London. The only interesting feature was the fellow travellers in boredom. On my right was a petite English woman who didn't give me the time of day, and on my left a very large – even by American standards – businessman who, no sooner was he settled into his seat after dinner, than he began snoring regularly and loudly. I opened a new Clancy novel, relishing five or six hours of pleasure, disturbed only by the unpleasant rumble. Whilst reading is no substitute for living, as many writers have reminded us, I love reading and never seem to have enough time. It's about the only way to enjoy an intimate intercourse with some very superior minds.

After several hours there was a hiatus in the snoring. The sudden absence of sound caught my attention, followed by a loud snort and a gross sucking sound as the contents of his sinuses were dragged down his throat as the American awoke. I focussed again on my book.

---

[*] A group of men from Kent in England who emigrated to New England in the Seventeenth Century.

'What you reading?' I was caught by surprise, so engrossed was I that I never realized my neighbour had actually woken.

'It's a new Clancy novel. I like his books.'

'Hmff, don't read myself.'

'Too bad. What line of business are you in?'

'I'm into lumber,' he growled. He had that lower octaves voice that the Americans seem to have perfected.

'Mm, that's a coincidence. I'm into lumbar too. Chiropractor or Orthopaedic surgeon?' *Let's see if this guy's awake yet,* I thought.

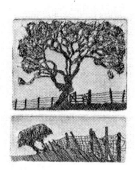

He looked at me blankly. 'What you talking about? I'm into lumber, you know, timber, trees. What do you do?'

'I'm a chiropractor. I work with lumbar, too. Wonky backs. I live in South Africa.'

'Oh yeah, South Africa. I have a friend who moved to a place called Lagos. You wouldn't know him would you? His name is Randy Elkington.'

'Well, actually no, I don't know him. Lagos is about five thousand miles from where I live. It's in Nigeria.' It never ceased to amaze me how little some Americans know about world geography. Was he thinking I would bump into his friend, 'Dr Livingstone, I presume' style?

'Is that a fact? Big place, South Africa.'

I didn't try to educate him. 'I do a lot of carpentry myself, but it's strictly recreational. Do you buy timber, sell it or grow it?' I gave a laugh.

'Naa, I sell it. Beech.'

'Mm, that's different. I've never worked with Beech before. Is it good wood to work with? What's the grain like?'

'No, we turn it into chips.'

'Ah, that's interesting. I like turning myself. Jacaranda is my favourite. This Superwood is an improvement, isn't it? Personally I can't stand that old chipboard. The screws never seem to hold.'

There was a slightly embarrassing silence and I was considering whether it would be rude to return to the Clancy.

'Actually, I sell it to the food industry.'

'Mm,' I said. 'Packaging, I suppose. Yes, it's good though plastics are taking over, aren't they? You can re-cycle wood products more easily, though.'

'No, not for packaging, the chips go into the food.'

I thought I had misunderstood. 'Whaa-t? Into the food? Who would want to put wood chips into food?'

'If you grind them up real fine, then they look just like the pips in strawberry jam.'

'Pips in strawberry jam? You must be joking, surely. What's wrong with the strawberry's own pips?'

'No, there are no strawberries in the jam they make. It's all imitation but it tastes real good.'

'Please, just run that by me again,' I said, my disbelief obvious.

'They take Halloween pumpkins, add red colouring and my wood chips for pips, then some sort of artificial sweetener so it's not fattening, and a strawberry flavouring. Hey, presto! You have strawberry jam.'

'I am a scientist and a Christian and on neither count can I bring myself to believe that, if you cross a pumpkin with a beech tree, you can get a strawberry,' I laughed. 'No matter how many times you wave the magic wand! Do they use genetic engineering?' I asked facetiously.

'No, none of that fancy stuff. Just plain old pumpkin, add my chips and some flavours and stuff and you've got beautiful jam. Some people prefer it to the real thing.'

'Hmff.' I was tiring of the conversation, deciding that I didn't care if I was rude. I returned to my book.

'You'll get to taste it with our breakfast – Atlantic Airlines is one of our big customers.'

I didn't look up.

If there's one thing I'm something of an expert on, it's strawberry jam. I sat back and closed my eyes thinking back of the days of agony. Early in our marriage when I was still a high school teacher, Helen and I had competitions to pick the strawberries she grew in abundance in her garden. Helen could pick at least three times as many and my poor ego suffered. In the early tussles for leadership in our marriage she was supposed to be the weaker sex, weaker at everything including strawberry picking; it wasn't for some long years that I began to appreciate the blessings that come with a strong wife. I blamed her superior strawberrying on her hypermobile back – Helen is one of those lucky women who can pick strawberries without bending her knees, but they can be something of a Chiropractic nightmare. My own back was already starting to creak and groan from all the beehives I had lifted so I picked strawberries while down on *one* knee. It's better than kneeling on both knees or squatting and certainly safer than bending.

Then came that day when the grade nine science class revealed all. We had just finished the study of spectrum colours, lenses and prisms, and the rods and cones in the human eye. The syllabus called for the section to be completed with a study of the Snellen chart for visual acuity and the Ishihara Test[*] for colour-blindness. I had never heard of them but it wasn't long before I was checking the boys for colour-blindness. Initially all went well through the various primary colours until I found the first boy with a defect: He saw a 5 where there was quite clearly a 2.

'Aha,' I exclaimed to the class, 'here we have a case of red/green colour blindness. Very interesting.' The boy paled.

---

[*] http://www.toledo-bend.com/colorblind/Ishihara.html

I called up the second boy. 'By George, he's also red/green colour blind!' And the third! Eventually it turned out that there were only two colour-blind people in that class. The teacher was one of them. In fact red-green colour blindness is quite common in boys, but very rare in girls. Helen had an unfair advantage.

Secretly, I was pleased; I was relegated to cutting and chopping the strawberries and stirring the pot when it threatened to boil over, while Helen tested the pectin and the gel point by placing drops on a plate into the freezer. We became quite a team and won a few prizes for the best strawberry jam at the Women's Institute Bake Sale. I know my strawberry jam.

The cabin lights came on and a stir rustled through the great monster as passengers were woken, started stretching and made their way towards the lavatory.

The English lady, too, woke. 'I hear you are a chiropractor. Can you tell me why people seem to stretch so naturally in the morning?'

I turned to her for the first time and noted her bright, intelligent eyes and engaging smile. Perhaps she was not so cold-hearted after all. Of course my mother was born into a very British family, so I knew all about the English stiff upper lip. 'Good morning. I wish everybody would stretch like that in the morning. Like many other important things, it's becoming increasingly lost in our modern, hurried society. There is hardly time for a good stretch.'

'Yes,' she said, pointing to a few of the passengers, 'but look at all those people.'

I sat for a moment, thinking, and wondering what to say. It was true that many of the passengers were stretching but, in my experience, very few of my patients stretch naturally. I have to instruct them how to do it. The thought came to mind, a gross over-simplification, of course, that perhaps *stretchers* are less likely to need a chiropractor, and my patients were made up mainly of the *non-stretchers* of the world.

'There are different reasons and no one simple answer. Just to give you two examples though, all the disc joints of the spine swell during the night so, if you don't stretch in the morning, you are more prone to injure your spine.'

'You mean we actually get taller?'

'Yes, that's true. Research on the people who have been in space has discovered that they return up to five centimetres taller. It's only temporary on Earth, of course. Under the effect of gravity, with the upright posture during the day, we get shorter again.'

'So that's quite normal then?'

'Yes, that's normal physiology.'

'Did they find anything else after space travel?'

'I am sure many things, but the only other one I am aware of related to health is that astronauts pass a lot of calcium in their urine.'

'Why is that?'

'At a guess, I would say it was due to the absence of weight-bearing inactivity. That's why women in particular must lead active lives. The alternative is broken bones when you get older.'

She nodded. 'A friend of mine broke her hip last month. She is only forty-eight.'

'That's because the authorities in their wisdom stopped compulsory school sport. There is now research clearly proving that children who play no sport are unlikely to have strong bones. I'm sure that is why middle-aged women have started breaking their hips.'

She didn't reply and I saw her, out of the corner of my eye, sitting proud and pondering all that. 'I suppose they thought they would be saving the country some money and could then lower taxes.'

'So instead you have obese and weak-boned children.'

'Bored ones too. And I suppose we end up paying out twice as much repairing hips and hearts.' She scowled. 'What was the other example?'

'Your muscles shorten during the night when they remain in the neutral position. Waste products build up in them and, unless you stretch them in the morning, they may become chronically shortened and prone to strain when you do something physical.'

'Like making the bed?' she asked.

'Or vacuuming the carpet,' I added. 'We may stretch a few muscles and joints like those people – I pointed to a few passengers who were still waking and stretching out an arm – but in my experience we don't do nearly enough of it, especially any joints and muscles that may have been injured in the past. That's where the focus of our stretching should be.'

'When you said "vacuuming" there was a tinge of malice in your voice.'

'I hate the vacuum cleaner. It's the chiropractor's greatest enemy! I can't tell you how many of my patients have been undone by the damned hoover!'

'Greatest enemy? Are you sure you don't mean greatest friend?' We laughed easily together.

The breakfast arrived and the lumberman went straight for the strawberry jam with a chuckle of excitement and anticipation. 'Here you are, just start with this,' he interrupted my conversation with the charming lady.

I opened the package of artificial looking airline food and took one small taste of the very realistic looking jam. I knew he was watching me in anticipation. Quietly I took the napkin and spat. 'I'm sorry,' I said, 'but I can't eat that. Anybody who has eaten as much real jam as I have, knows that your so-called strawberry jam tastes just like woodpulp and Halloween witches and I'm not too partial to either, first thing in the morning. Carpentry after lunch and pumpkin for dinner!' I tried to make a joke of it but he was offended.

'Hmph,' he grunted, and never said another word to me for the rest of the trip.

My maternal cousin was in Terminal Four to meet me. We embraced and I found myself quite emotional. He had left South Africa at the height of the Apartheid era when young white men were expected to join the army for two years and enforce that evil social system. George and I had been best friends as kids. We had sat under Nana's fruit trees during our holidays and munched our way through six mangoes and a dozen *litchis,*[*] filling our hollow legs, before the serious part of breakfast had even started. We had fished together, hiked the Drakensberg mountains, discussed our first girlfriends, and his decision to emigrate had been very hurtful to us both. Our friendship had been abruptly amputated.

There was a lot of ground to cover and the drive to Kent was animated once we had broken the ice of two decades. I enjoyed the scenery, glancing out the window at the sheep and the rows of hops surrounded by hedgerows, quite different from New England. There were road signs ahead and I noticed 'Brenchley's Green'. 'George, can we pop in there for a moment? Is it far from the road?'

He swung off the highway and we meandered down narrow English lanes while I told him the story of Ebenezer Preston. I found it astonishing how the English park their cars in the road, and we had to stop periodically as the road narrowed to one lane but the English appear to be the most patient nation on Earth. I had difficulty holding my tongue, thinking of the wide roads in the land of our birth.

Not far from the M20 we found the little village with its ancient stone church. After parking under a row of Yews, we walked down some very old, worn stone steps to the vestry door but the whole church was firmly locked.

---

[*] Delicious tropical fruit.

'There's the cemetery,' George called, pointing.

We strolled nonchalantly through a creaking old gate. George glanced at me doubtfully as we were confronted by a graveyard filled with ancient tombstones, many of them more than two hundred years old, covered with moss and lichen and quite illegible. Where to start?

'Can I help you?' an old man called, the verger, I presumed.

'I'm looking for the tombstone of an Ebenezer Preston. Where do you suggest we start?'

'Och aye, Ebenezer's over in that corner.' He gestured down the cemetery towards the lower end where the oldest stones lay. The old man hung about ingratiating himself to us, which was fortunate. We would never have found Ebenezer's grave without his help. The stone had an unusual double top and the name was virtually illegible. I sat in front of the stone, rubbing out the lichen and gradually the letters became clearer. 'George, come and look at this,' I shouted, unable to keep the excitement from my voice. 'This is unbelievable!'

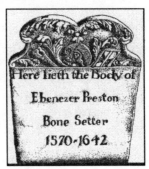

Here lieth the Body of
Ebenezer Preston
Bone Setter
1570-1642

'What's a bone-setter, Bernie?'

'George, my great, great, dozens of greats, grandfather was the first edition of a chiropractor.'

Chapter Thirteen

GREED

Often patient satisfaction is not so much driven by the doctor's technical expertise as by the patient's feeling of being cared about.

Dr Robert Shiel

Life is not inherently fair, at least not from our human perspective. Some people, *poor* people we would say, seem to get a double portion of pain. Danny McFie was one of them. I had known the McFies for some years, not particularly well as they were fortunate enough to have healthy bodies or, at least, so we thought.

'Been sitting too much in front of your computer again, Danny?' I asked during one such consultation, not long after my extended American holiday.

'Yes, I guess, Doc.'

'And has your skipping-rope[*] been stolen or just neglected?'

I knew Danny wouldn't mind me pulling his leg. Theft was what gave him a job. He was an electronic engineer who had made considerable mileage out of South Africa's grand auto theft industry. The word *grand* described it very adequately. In a society of such contrast between have and have-nots, car theft was deemed by some to be a legitimate way to redistribute wealth in the new South Africa. It was Danny's company that discovered a niche market: electronic devices to make the thief's work a lot more difficult. Such

---

[*] Jump rope.

was Danny's prowess that the company became a world leader in the design and manufacture of such devices. One of the things that makes the practice of Chiropractic so interesting is the insight into people's lives that comes while I am at work on their spines.

He laughed. 'Just neglected. Now that winter is coming on, it's dark when I get home in the evening and I don't feel like exercising.'

'Come on, Danny. That's just the time when the rope comes into its own. During the summer you should be taking to the pool or playing a set or two of tennis with Sharon after work. Winter is skipping-rope season.'

I'm a great believer in the skipping-rope. Gyms don't turn many people on and some don't have the money for a gym contract. Danny did have the money but, like me I might say, just didn't have the time or the inclination; but we all need exercise in a society where we sit far too much. The skipping-rope is the busy man's total body workout in ten minutes.

'How's business?' I asked, changing the direction of our conversation, not wanting to be a fishwife. I had made my point and there was no need to belabour it. Danny fortunately had a very healthy back and had only the odd episode of low back pain that responded very quickly to half a dozen spinal adjustments and a set of exercises. When he did them, that is.

'Fantastic! We've just landed a contract to supply the total world-wide market with anti-hijacking devices for a large German manufacturer. It will be worth millions.'

'That's amazing. Congratulations. And how are Sharon and Tamsin?'

'Oh, I wish Sharon would sell her dry-cleaning business. We don't need the money any more, and now that Tamsin has turned fourteen, she's needing a mother when she gets home from school. The boys are starting to take an interest and that gets me nervous. I don't know who her husband will be but, already, I dislike him!'

'That's quite normal, Danny, even more so seeing that she's your only child. Just get the shot-gun loaded with salt,' I laughed.

Danny's first portion of pain struck about six months later. Sharon was diagnosed with leukaemia, ostensibly from the nasty chemicals that dry-cleaners are exposed to. Danny seemed to need more treatment for his back during the months that followed so I knew something of his misery.

'Doc, would you consider becoming a tissue donor?' Danny asked me one afternoon. He knew that I visited the vampires periodically and they were searching in vain for a suitable donor of bone marrow stem cells. I didn't match but it was good to have joined the register of donors. Maybe one day my blood would match someone else in need.

Danny loved to tease me. He always parked his convertible directly outside my office window. It was a dark green colour which matched my mood and my envy. One day I watched him struggling to get out of the low sports car. 'Serves you right, Danny, for always parking it where you know I can see it.'

'With only one pair of hands, you'll never earn enough money to buy one of the topless ladies, Doc, but just in case you win the lottery, the French are making really good sports cars for about half the price of the Germans and Italians. Perhaps I'll design a robot that can give manipulations and then you can treat dozens of people simultaneously!'

Nine months later I watched Danny struggle out of a battered old Beetle that he had parked in his usual spot. He limped down to my office with more than his usual pain. I was concerned, not only because of Sharon, but because this was definitely a more serious episode than his usual mild sacro-iliac strain. And the car? After I had completed my examination, I asked him to sit for a moment which he did with some difficulty. 'Danny, most of the orthopaedic tests point to a SI strain, which is what you usually have.'

'Tell me again, Doc. What's an SI? Sorry, I know you've explained it all before.'

'It's this joint between the sacrum and the ilium,' I said, demonstrating to him on my very precious old dry spine. 'SIJ for Sacro-Iliac joint.'

'Is that plastic?' he asked, looking at the spine.

'No, she was a real Indian lady. India has so many unclaimed bodies that they made an industry of it, exporting spines to the world. She's very special and I have a sense of being on hallowed ground every time I touch her. But to return to your back: As we have discussed before, SI strain can lead to injury to the disc. I'm afraid today you have a strongly positive *Slump test*,[*] so I want you to take three days of bed rest. Do these three exercises every half an hour, and every hour get up and go for a short walk around the house. Make a cup of tea, have a pee, you know, just get onto your feet.'

'Why is it important to get up, Doc? It hurts so much to get out of bed and it literally took me nearly five minutes just to pluck up the courage to lie down again!'

'During prolonged lying down, the injured joint swells, Danny. All the research shows that extended bed rest is not helpful, but I find that the rest coupled with these exercises, and getting up periodically, is what helps. Use an ice pack twice a day for half an hour, followed by a little heat, please.'

We went through the exercises carefully again. I had to be sure that he did them correctly and that they were suitable.

'Did you design these exercises, Doc?'

'Actually Danny, a physiotherapist by the name of Williams gets the credit, but I'm sure the ancient Egyptians were doing them about five millennia BW.'

'BW?' He looked at me blankly.

'Before Williams. Sorry, that's a bit corny!'

---

[*] An orthopaedic test for a pinched nerve.

'You don't mind using exercises credited to a physio?' Danny laughed. He was regaining his sense of humour.

'I'll use anything that helps you, Danny. Physio, acupuncture, massage, even medication or surgery if it's necessary. It's your health, not my philosophy of care that counts.'

The next day Danny was a little better. While I was working on his back, I again noticed the battered old Beetle parked where the BMW usually sat, provoking my envy. 'What's happened to the car, Danny?'

Danny was silent for a while. I gave him space. 'The medical insurance would only pay for Sharon's treatment for twelve months. We're now having to find the money for her chemo. The M3 had to go.'

'That's a shame. You'll get another one in time. Bigger and better. Maybe smaller and better?'

He ignored that. I could see he was struggling with something. 'Doc, could we talk about something that's been bothering me?'

'Go ahead.'

'Once our medical insurance ran out, the attitude of the oncologist towards Sharon changed. He just said, "Well, there's not much more we can do now." It was almost that now he couldn't make any more money out of us, he lost interest.'

'Didn't you tell him about your topless Italian lady that you were selling?'

'Yes, I did, but the bank owned that car anyway. Most of the saving was in the insurance that I had to pay. That insurance was enough to keep a poor man in a luxurious life style!' he said, with a fragile grin.

'This whole thing of the money is one we all struggle with, Danny. I know when I started in practice, I didn't want to take people's money so I would discharge them long before they were better. Then I swung towards greed when I wanted to buy my first glider, and tried to squeeze an extra treatment or two out of my patients. It took quite a long time to reach higher ground: that place where you take your eyes off the dollar signs and do what you have to do.'

After one year, through some fine print in the contract, the insurance company refused further medical payments. Quite rapidly Danny was stripped of all his wealth. First he had to sell his fancy car, and then their house went on the market. Sharon was a fighter, not wanting her daughter to go through the formative all-important teenage years without a mother, but first the chemotherapy and the prolonged radiation, and then the bone marrow transplant impoverished them.

'Doc, my back's nearly better, do you mind if we miss the last few treatments?' Danny knew how much store I placed by the proper rehabilitation of spinal injuries. 'I'm sorry, but I just don't have the money for your treatment, and I think I know what to do.'

I weighed his request carefully. Should I offer free treatment? Or place the extra responsibility on his own shoulders? He did indeed know what was needed but would he do it?

'Okay, Danny, just remember that it will be at least two weeks before you can trust your back. Those exercises must go on at least twice a day, and please try not to sit too much yet, particularly in the car or on the lounge furniture.'

Danny nodded, looking away. I was saddened to see how the first bite of poverty had reduced his usual ebullient self. Life was stripping off his protective layers, leaving him vulnerable and naked.

'Will you phone me in a week?' I always like to keep control until I know the patient is well. Too often one sneeze or some foolishness starts things up again.

Danny got better, as he always did, in a few weeks. But Sharon didn't. Danny phoned me periodically, just to chat, so I knew of his wife's slow decline as her body rejected the new bone marrow. They never found a perfect match. The funeral was a sad affair.

Danny's second portion of pain was much worse. Fortunately, Sharon was spared the agony. About a year after her death Danny arrived home one evening, finding a dark and silent house. That happened periodically, but Tamsin always phoned him to ask if she could stay with a friend or go to a movie. By nine o'clock he started to worry and began phoning friends. 'Have you seen Tamsin?' But none of her friends knew anything of her whereabouts. By midnight Danny was panicking. He had phoned Tamsin's boyfriend and all the hospitals, and the police had put out photos and her description to the newspapers. ANOTHER TEENAGER GONE AWOL. Nothing unusual about that, the police told him. They had reports of them all the time.

When I saw Tamsin's photo on the front page of the *East Griqualand Herald*, I picked up the phone. 'Any news, Danny?'

'None, Doc. Absolutely nothing.'

'I'm sure the police have asked you, but was everything between you okay?'

'Yes, absolutely normal.'

'If there's anything I can do to help please let me know, Danny.'

'Sure, Doc.' I could hear he was in tears.

Tamsin was never found. She just vanished from the planet. About a year later the police attempted to arrest a paedophile in East London. He first shot his girlfriend accomplice and then blew his own brains out, taking the secret of Tamsin and at least five other girls with them into eternity. They found Tamsin's purse in his house.

The phone rang one Saturday evening as I drove in the gate from soaring. Helen passed me the phone. 'Hello, Bernie Preston,' I said.

'Hi Doc, this is Danny.'

'Hello, Danny. Any news?'

'Yes, Doc. Can I come up and chat? Would you mind?'

'Of course, Danny. Do you know where we live in High Whytten?'

'Yes, I'll be there in half an hour, if that's okay?'

With only himself to care for, relative wealth had returned to Danny's life. He had no inclination for another 'topless lady' but the battered old Beatle was gone. He arrived in a good second-hand Honda Ballade.

Helen made us coffee and we sat out on the veranda. Being stuck indoors for so many hours of the week, I prefer the outdoors to the TV room. I also have a strong suspicion that when they come to write the 'Rise and Fall' of this civilization, TV will be one of the main causes of its demise. In any case it's much better to have fun yourself than watch others enjoying themselves. That evening with Danny wasn't fun, though.

'Still no sign of Tamsin, I presume.'

He sighed: 'Nope, she's gone for ever. I'm sure she's dead.'

I didn't know what to say, so I said nothing. Eventually after another cup of coffee and a piece of Helen's fruit cake covered with a dollop of ice cream, Danny said: 'I've had an offer for a job in New Hampshire and I think I'm going to take it. What do you think?'

'Too many bad memories here,' I said. 'If I was you I would go for it. I was born there strangely enough.'

'You were born in New Hampshire! That's a coincidence. What's it like?'

'Beautiful,' I said. 'It's the big outdoors with dozens of lakes, and forests and ski resorts. Breath taking. Very cold in the winter, of course.'

There was a silence for a while. 'My only worry is if somehow Tamsin should show up, or call for help or something. I know she won't, but I just feel I can't go off and not leave something behind. Would you mind terribly if I put my phone through to your house for a year? I would pay for it, of course. And keep your ears open.' He looked at me, pleading, anguish in his eyes.

'Of course, Danny. I would be absolutely delighted to help in any way I can. When you know you're going, give me a call and I'll write a report for a chiropractor in the States. That way he won't have to reinvent the wheel. We already know what pattern of adjustments and exercises work for your back.'

Within three months Danny was gone. He got his report and his x-rays which were almost new, and I got an extra phone line. It had its uses in those early internet days. I had the odd email from him but, of course, there was no sign of Tamsin.

Nearly a year passed when I received a frantic email from Danny:

Hey, Doc, could you advise me. I've started getting a few twinges in my back, so I went to the chiro in Charter's Creek. It was no big deal but I thought I had better go before it got bad. I gave him your report and the x-rays. He gave me a thorough examination and insisted on a new set of full spine x-rays. In his report of findings, he then proceeded to tell me what serious problems I had in my spine. I would need to go to him three times a week for three months, and then once a week for 9 months. It seems an awful lot of treatment, and I'm not even really sore. In fact, with your exercises and that one treatment, I feel fifty per cent better. At the next consultation I have to sign a contract for a whole year. It sounds bogus to me, but I thought I would ask what you thought.
Regards,
Danny.

Charter's Creek! What a coincidence; precisely where I was born and where most of my American family still lived.

I did a quick calculation:

3 months x 4 wks x 3 treatments per week = 36.

Add to that:

9 months x 4 weeks x 1 treatment per week = another 36.

72 manipulations in a year! Times about $40. Nearly $3000!

Medicine has been honest and openly admitted that the frequent use of antibiotics amounts to abuse. Not that some doctors are not still overly enthusiastic with their prescription pads, but at least as a profession they have begun to be more cautious. Antibiotics have saved millions of lives but over-prescription has killed a good many too.

As a much younger profession, we have not yet come to the place of defining how much manipulation is 'too much manipulation'. Some chiropractors don't even think there is such a thing. Research on the amount of Chiropractic care needed is now beginning to trickle in but one thing I knew: Danny was being ripped off, and his spine was about to be abused. It was little wonder my family wouldn't consult their local chiropractor. Danny's instincts were absolutely correct.

Dear Danny

I'm sorry to have to say this, but under no circumstances go back or sign anything. If you have paid for the x-rays, go and collect them.

Then I would suggest you start to ask around. None of us in the healing world have a perfect record but you will quite quickly find the people will start saying: this guy is good, or stay away from that woman, for one reason or another. Follow your instincts as you did this time.

In this hemisphere, no news is bad news, I'm afraid. Not a word about Tamsin. I have taken over the payment of your phone. The extra line has come in very useful.

Let me know how you get on with the next chiropractor!

Regards

Bernie.

I got a reply from Danny some weeks later.

Thanks for the advice. I found a fantastic lady chiropractor in the next town. I'm fine and you won't believe it: every night when I get home it's pitch black, so I do ten minutes of skipping!

The good chiropractor has to be something of a fish-wife, something of a bully, and something of a confidant and friend. Not an easy balance to find. Then it goes without saying that you miss some patients, thinking about them long after they die, or emigrate.

That's great, Danny. Please let me have her name. My family also lives in Charter's Creek and they are desperately in need of a good chiropractor.

It was another five years, on a visit to my American family, before I connected with Danny again. He had married a widow with three children. They had a lovely home on the lake and we enjoyed a beautiful cruise in the boat that he kept at the dock just in front of their home. I noticed there was another topless lady parked 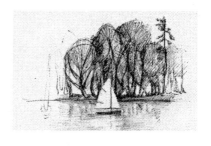 outside their home. Yellow, befitted his mood these days apparently, rather than the olive green that still suited mine.

Chapter Fourteen

GET YOUR OWN BACK…

The voice of conscience is so delicate that it is easy to stifle it; but it is also so clear that it is impossible to mistake it.

Madame De Stael

I did not know Karin well as a patient – she had only been in a few times over a two-year period – but I knew enough to know that something was seriously wrong. Something that had nothing to do with the pain in her back.

A very attractive 'life and soul of the party' girl, she had consulted me a few times for the sorts of aches and pains that people who sit for long hours hunched over a computer experience. Fortunately she was also a dancer and that brought balance to her life, though it also brought its share of 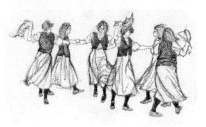 pulled muscles and sprained joints in the lower limbs. Latin was her speciality, but she supplemented her meagre salary by dancing the maypole or the can-can in the local mall on Saturday mornings.

Karin wasn't a dumb blonde, but she never got out of the typing pool for some reason. I had expected her to aim higher. It was however her bubbling personality that made her really attractive. Now, all that was gone and every time I touched her she flinched.

'When did this pain begin, Karin?' I started. She had pain right down the left side of her back. It was quite unusual. Later, during the examination, I found that not only did she have multiple sprained joints throughout her back, *subluxations* we call them, but also orthopedic testing showed equal signs of muscular strain.

'About two months ago,' was all I got. She wouldn't give me any details.

'This has nothing to do with your dancing?' She shook her head.

At the next consultation she finally admitted that she had been in a fight. It did make sense. There were still some signs of fading bruises; they must have been bad at the time.

Spinal x-rays showed nothing, and still I knew she was holding something back. Every time I touched her unexpectedly, she gave an involuntary flinch. I started with the usual sort of treatment: I gently adjusted the injured joints – she was in a lot of pain – then stretched and did some cross friction on the muscles of her back and right shoulder. Karin then had a series of daily massages by a masseuse we employ in the clinic followed by fifteen minutes in the pool. Finally, after a few weeks, to complete my programme which was geared at treating her physical injuries, I asked her to either go cycling or jogging for half an hour. Karin's body healed, but despite that, she still flinched if I walked into the consulting room, or touched her, unexpectedly.

'Are you ready to tell me what really happened?' I asked suddenly one day, not long before she was ready for discharge. She no longer had pain in the back, but her bubbling personality showed no signs of returning.

Karin began to cry, putting her hands over her face and, finally between her fingers, cried out: 'The bastard raped me, and now I'm pregnant.' The whimpering turned into loud, deep sobs as the deep, unacknowledged pain of the last three months came bursting out. 'I just can't make the decision – am I going to abort the baby, or not?' I put my arms around her, consoling her, and beginning to understand something of her anguish. Who could understand it all? She wasn't much older than my own daughter. I shuddered at the thought.

'Like a fool I went home with a guy after a rave at a city night club. We were having such a good time, and it was much too late to phone my dad to fetch me. I was such a fool. Once he had me in his home we kissed and cuddled a little and then he raped me. I pleaded with him to stop, but he just went on and on. It was horrible.' There were more bouts of uncontrolled sobbing.

'Who is he? Did you lay a charge against him?'

'It would be no good. No one would believe me. I went to his home of my own free will. My friends saw me getting quite happily into his car. His name is Tom Phipson, he's the lover boy of the night club scene. Lots of girls would love to get into his bed, but I wasn't ready for it. I'm not that sort, but he wouldn't stop.'

'Has he done it before? What do the other girls say?'

She nodded. 'There are lots of rumours but nobody will come out and say anything and so he goes on. He knows we won't squeal. I'm going to stop him but I don't know how.'

I thought for a while. 'You have two choices: take him to court, and yes you are right, you will have difficulty getting a conviction. It might tarnish his name, but it probably won't stop him.'

'And the other?'

'You could try and humiliate him publicly.'

'How would I do that?'

'Give me some time to think about it? I'll come up with an answer. You think about it too.'

What made Karin's story particularly painful was that she had committed her life to Christ just a month before she was raped. How could God allow such a thing to happen to one of His newly adopted daughters? I had a heavy heart.

My first patient the next morning was a Black Belt karate champion. An awesome kick in the small of his back at the World Games some six months earlier had fractured a small isthmus of bone in his back called the *Pars Interarticularis.*[*] Normally that fracture only happens in childhood when the bone hasn't set, in fact some think it's congenital. Pete was one of the few adult patients that I had treated with a fresh Pars fracture. I had him in a corset for three months and surprisingly the fracture was healing. He had been smart and consulted me the day he got back from the Games. He knew that he had done himself a mischief.

'Pete, could you teach a young woman to slap a guy in public really hard before he had time to react?'

'Easy,' said Pete, 'unless he is also trained in martial arts. No problem.'

I gave Karin a call: 'Come to the clinic at lunch time tomorrow. I have some ideas.' Next day I explained to Karin that the first part would be several weeks of training from a karate champ called Pete van Dijk. She was just beginning to show signs of her pregnancy, but Karin took to the idea and went into the training enthusiastically.

Pete phoned me three weeks later: 'I think she's ready, Doc, but it could go all wrong. We need to plan this carefully.'

'I'll come down to the gym at about six this evening. Make sure Karin's there and we'll go through the strategy.'

When I arrived I was astonished by the depth of training in the gym, the absolute commitment I could see on their faces, and yet it remained, in the main, a non-contact sport. The trick was to pull your punch or your kick one millimetre short of your opponent's nose. Karin and Pete were there to greet me. Karin had found such a sense of achievement out of

---

[*] Small piece of bone in the spine that is sometimes fractured in trauma, leading to instability of the spine and, frequently chronic low back pain.

her training that she had joined the gym and was in the same leotard as all the other women, despite beginning to show unmistakable signs of her pregnancy. We went over into a corner.

'So how are you going to engineer the end of this lover-boy's free sex life?' I asked.

'We decided on something very simple: Pete and a couple of his friends come up behind him, just in case things go wrong, and I walk up to him, smile sweetly, and clobber him. He won't be expecting it,' Karin said.

'Yes, that would work but it won't really achieve what you set out to do, and that was to humiliate him in front of a lot of people. Probably no more than half a dozen people will see it. You want every woman in the club to witness it. It wouldn't do any harm for the men also to see what can happen to a guy who rapes girls.'

'How am I going to do that?' she asked.

I thought for a moment. 'You don't by any chance know the owner of the club, do you?'

She shook her head but Pete came to the rescue. 'I could easily go and ask him to do me a favour.'

'That's perfect,' I said, but now you've got to practise it, again and again. You will only get one chance.'

We were talking over a few more details when I had another thought. 'Karin, go in a maternity dress. Add a few layers and make it very obvious you are pregnant. If you're dancing with Pete somewhere near Mister Tom Phipson, I guarantee he will come over to investigate his handiwork. That will be your cue. Pete, you must be sure you have a couple of pals nearby, and one on the mike.'

The trap couldn't have worked better. Karin figured that Tom wouldn't remember exactly when he had raped her, as she hadn't seen him since that night. Her friends gathered around her excitedly wanting to know about the baby. That set the bait perfectly. She danced away the evening with Pete while a friend hovered near the mike for his cue.

Sure enough, a little after eleven, just as the music was getting louder and the beat more insistent, Tom Phipson could not resist his curiosity any longer. He wanted to find out more about his baby.

'Well, well, well, what do we have here?' he leered at her, reaching out his hand to rub her belly. She pushed his hands away.

'Keep your hands off me, Tom,' Karin said.

Just then the music stopped and, very suddenly, a loud voice announcing over the PA system: 'Listen up everybody. Karin over here has something important to say.' He pointed in her direction, and everybody's gaze swept over to the couple. Tom was momentarily distracted.

'Hello everybody,' Karin called out as loud as she could. The club was quiet for once. Somebody held a portable mike near her. 'As you all can see I am very pregnant, and Tom here is the father.' There were some cheers and wolf-whistles and Tom took his eyes off Karin looking for his fans. Before he knew it, Karin had walloped him hard with her right hand, and then with her left fist. Tom took the punch on the nose, knocking him off balance, for a moment. A couple of Pete's friends quickly grabbed his arms and Karin shouted out: 'He raped me, the bastard, and now I am HIV positive. Stay away from him, girls.'

Pete phoned the next day: 'It went well, Doc. Planned and executed with precision. I do think you could have told me though, that Karin is HIV positive.' He was angry.

'Oh, no! Why didn't she tell me, poor girl?'

'You didn't know?'

'Not at all,' I replied.

Karin popped in at lunch time to tell me all about it. She had regained all her enthusiasm and bounce, but all I could think of was HIV, those three nasty letters that make up a death sentence.

'Why didn't you tell me?'

'Tell you what?'

'That he also infected you with HIV.'

She laughed out aloud. 'He didn't. I just added that for spice. And for spite!'

'You're still going to have the baby?'

She looked at me for long moments, a little smile creeping first from her eyes, through to the corners of her mouth. She nodded: 'Yes, I'm going to have this baby. I had an exam from my gynae, Dr Simmons, this morning and that confirmed it.'

'Oh?'

She nodded again. 'He told me about a couple who have been consulting him for a few months. They have been trying for ten years to have a baby, but the man's sperm count is virtually non-existent. He had been kicked *you know where* in a rugby match.

'And?'

'He said they were the nicest people, and' – she sniffed, and smiled – 'would make the best possible parents for my baby. They would even pay for the whole confinement.'

Things did work out ultimately for Karin's good, but for many months there was heart ache and drama. Pete was one of the good things. The final twist in that tale, though, many years later, brought tears to *my* eyes.

Appendix 1 to Chapter Fourteen

125 Rondebosch Road
Cape Town

Dear Dr Simmons,

I'm sure you won't remember me as the events mentioned here occurred nearly a quarter of a century ago, and I expect have been repeated many times in your practice.

I write to thank you for encouraging me not to have an abortion. Three months ago I received the phone call that every mother who gives up her baby for adoption waits for. It went something like this:

'Is that Mrs van Dijk?'

'Uh, ye-es. Who is this?'

'Um, this is Emily Stratford. I am phoning from Boston in the United States. I'll get right to the point, Mrs van Dijk. Did you once have a daughter that you gave up for adoption? About 25 years ago?'

I'll admit there was a long silence here. I didn't know how to answer. The call that I had been expecting for so long, suddenly was the unexpected.

'Are you there Mrs van Dijk?'

'Yes, yes I am here. Yes, Emily, were you born on August 12th?'

Well, Dr Simmons, Emily is indeed my daughter. I have just returned from a wonderful trip to her wedding in America. After the phone call, she asked if she and her fiancé could visit me. They came first and foremost to thank me for not aborting her. What followed was a trip to her family home in Connecticut for the wedding.

I have three younger children and now, thanks to your advice, the great blessing of a fourth.

In deep appreciation of your wisdom and care.

Yours very sincerely

(Mrs) Karin van Dijk.

Appendix 2 to Chapter Fourteen

125 Rondebosch Road
Cape Town

Dear Dr Preston

I enclose herein a copy of a self-explanatory letter to Dr Simmons. I like to think that you might remember me, Dr Preston, although the events described here occurred a long time ago.

I came to you for treatment for a sore back. You helped me to expose the horrible man who raped me by introducing me to Pete van Dijk, a karate champion. Do you remember the visits to Pete's gym, and the strategy planning? Not long after the birth of my daughter, Pete and I started dating and, soon after we married, we moved to Cape Town to escape the memories of Shafton.

It was wonderful to meet my daughter, and I thank you deeply for the part you played in helping me get through the rape ordeal, and of course introducing me to the most wonderful man.

If ever you come to come to Cape Town... please pay us a visit.

Yours sincerely

Karin van Dijk.

Chapter Fifteen

BAPTISO – TO IMMERSE

Success is not the key to happiness.
Happiness is the key to success.

Albert Schweitzer

I was first baptised, aged three months, *into a pagan family* so it didn't really count. The bishops didn't approve of my theology when, at the second visit to the font I was baptised, aged nineteen, *into Christ*. The third time? In my dotage, *into humility*. It happened one Saturday like this.

I woke early and went out into the garden for a sweet pee. A half moon and Venus were in close proximity, brilliantly etched against the eastern sky, greeting each other as it were. A scattering of cumulus, brilliantly white in the early dawn stretched westwards, fading as the clouds further west still desperately avoided the probing rays of the as yet invisible burning sun. All was silhouetted against a blue-black sky. *Could be a good day*, I mused. Glider pilots are inveterate optimists, gazing hopefully into the heavenlies every Saturday morning. It was one of those magical moments that only the *'early to bed, early to rise'* devotees can enjoy. By the time Helen rises from her beauty sleep the best part of the day is already done! The crisp early African morning has a beauty that never seems to cloy, and in me there is a deep appreciation of a life that does not dull, despite ten thousand similar dawns. No, today's was different. I couldn't recall even one that was vaguely like it.

A stroll in the garden definitely beats the toilet for relieving yourself first thing in the morning, I thought, with only a few *Hadedas* to squawk at me. The Cymbidiums were beginning to spike and they needed the extra urea, I reasoned.

I picked up the *East Griqualand Herald* at the gate, going through the daily struggle; *shall I read the Good News or the Bad News first?* Three mugs of tea later both my soul and my need to keep up to date with world events were satisfied and I started preparing for what was to be *the day*. I was still blissfully ignorant, of course. Ahead lay a day that would remain indelibly etched on my mind for the rest of my life. Batteries for the radios were on charge, hats packed, tea and some home-made bread were all in readiness. I hurriedly pared a cucumber for fibre and sliced a tomato for my prostate, all in vain. None would be eaten. Had I been able to look into the crystal ball I would have saved myself the trouble. It was just as well that I had fully charged those batteries, though. I was going to need them.

It's a funny thing, the earlier I rise, the later I get going. I was late in arriving at the gliding club that day but then I did have to spend a few hours at the clinic. My patients that morning included an elderly lady with a very painful neck after being savagely beaten by intruders, a couple of routine sore backs and a young man with a fracture in his spine after a car accident. I updated all the day's files, so that I could leave the clinic with a good conscience, and completed the detailed report for the lawyer. He was determined that his client would be fully recompensed by the Road Accident Fund, and his cut too of course which, in the gospel according to Abba, makes the world go round: Money, money, money... Do we acquire our fortunes or do they ensnare us?

It was not to be a routine day, either at the clinic or later in my favourite pastime. I should have guessed right then that something remarkable in the sky was awaiting me.

The dash to the club was also memorable. I was late, and now even later. As I approached the airfield I was stopped at the site of a minibus taxi lying on its side, dead bodies strewn about the road. Fortunately the ambulance and the police had already arrived. Unable to stop myself staring at the carnage, my mind travelled down an old familiar track, having difficulty taking off the Chiropractic hat and putting on my soaring cap: The so-called road *accidents* that brought me so much work should really be named road *trauma;* they are after all no accident, being in the main highly predictable and it is going to take rather more than a few feeble clichés like 'Zero tolerance' that soft-headed politicians like to promote to stop the terrible suffering on South African roads.

I allowed my mind to drift as I drove on to the club, trying to forget my responsibilities as a chiropractor and the mayhem I had just witnessed, which was perhaps a good thing. That mind was going to be extremely focussed for the rest of the day as I struggled to stamp my authority on the elements, denying them their natural inclination to punish those who dare to defy them.

Late arrivees are sent straight to the winch that launches our gliders into the sky and so I did my penance. 'Don't apologise,' said Carl, one of our best instructors, with a smile. 'We love it when you get here late. Then there's no fuss about who is going to be on the winch. You!' he finished, poking me on the chest. Being stuck on the ground is not a pilot's idea of fun.

So the next couple hours were spent launching my friends' gliders and, for once, events turned out well for the latecomer. The gliders all fell out of the sky as the elements retained the early upper hand. An early launch would have been in vain. I smirked, watching a street of clouds developing, reaching out towards the north-west. This might be a good day yet.

Finally the next winch driver arrived. 'There is only very strong sink, Bernie,' Shirley said. 'Don't stray too far from the airfield or you might find yourself out-landing!' Glider pilots are not all male. There are also a few women, equally intrepid or mad, according to your viewpoint, smitten by soaring.

'When there's strong sink, Shirley, there's also strong lift. I'm going to find it!'

'Yes, yes, Bernie, the eternal optimist, always arrogant. I give you no more than ten minutes aloft.' Shirley smiled at me as we swapped places and I drove over to the clubhouse to haul out my ancient Ka6 from its hangar. A new member who wanted to please lent a helping hand.

In fact, I was wrong. It was Shirley's husband in his beautiful ASW 15, a fibreglass ship that stood out in sharp contrast to my old plywood crate, who found the lift.

'Turn round, Bernie, and fly straight back to the launch point. There's a beautiful *blue thermal** over the copse of Wattle trees,' Graham called on the radio from aloft while I was preparing for take-off. Thermals are often marked by a cloud but blue thermals were found simply by luck. Graham had the first dip into the lucky-packet. I craned my head, scanning the sky for his glider from my tiny cramped space in the cockpit, feeling a tiny crick in my neck. *Ah, there he is*, I could see Graham above my head banking steeply and, even from the ground, I could see that his glider was climbing fast. *Hooray! Big boys and their toys,* I taunted myself, recognizing a still present need for childlike excitement.

Shirley gave me a beautiful launch with the needle hovering around 90kph and, when I pulled the release cable, I found myself at 1400 feet agl (*above ground level*). The altimeter, of course, gave me the height *above sea level*, 6,000 feet asl. I checked my speed and turned sharply back to where I had seen Graham's glider. He was already at least 2000 feet above me, but there was very strong sink all the way back to the invisible thermal. I was sinking fast and gave

---

* Thermal found under a blue sky (with no white cloud marking the top of the thermal.

a groan when I found myself at 600 feet above ground and having to prepare for a landing circuit. Then the variometer started to sing and I felt the *big hand* smack me in the seat of the pants. I waited the customary three seconds so as not to fly right through the thermal and then banked steeply, using the ailerons and adjusting the rudder pedals. The first turn saw me climb a hundred feet or so and my groan turned to a shout of exultation. *Up, up and away.* Within fifteen minutes my glider carried me all the way to ten thousand feet above sea level in one beautiful thermal.

I was joined by a pair of giant Secretarybirds. Like gliders they are stiff and ungainly on the ground but, with a wing-span approaching one and half metres, they are astonishingly elegant in the air. From the vantage point of my cockpit I watched them playing the giddy-goat, fooling about with each other. Thermalling one moment just off my wing tips and then diving and swooping, by dropping their legs for airbrakes in a most odd manner, they were quite unperturbed by their giant white companion. I sighed, supremely contented. Eventually the birds, bored of my company, dived and I watched them land in the centre of the runway nearly two kilometres below, disturbing proceedings on the ground. It was a divine moment.

Cloud base was another 2,000 feet above my head but the ceiling of our airspace over the club was restricted to 10,000 feet above sea level. I was not allowed to soar any higher here. I watched Graham turn and fly over Lake Msimang, leaving the restricted area and heading further north towards the great dam wall. He hit the strong sink and I decided to go further south towards a promising looking cloud with a dark-grey underbelly. It was the right decision. Graham never got back to 10,000 feet and we had to shelve our plan to investigate the Midlands, west of the airfield, together. I too hit the sink but, on the far side of the lake, over Mount Aston, having sunk to 8,000 feet I found the thermal of the day. I was now outside the gliding window that had restricted me to

10,000 feet and my glider soared even higher into the sky. I gave a little shiver, a pleasurable frisson of anticipation. Or was it just the cold? At launch the cockpit thermometer had read forty-two degrees Celsius in my little greenhouse. I watched as it plunged down to ten degrees, a jet of cold air turning my nose red. I stuffed an old handkerchief into the aperture in the Perspex canopy, pulled my cap a little deeper over my head and wished I had a scarf.

'Yankee Zulu, this is Alpha X-ray. What's happening, Graham?' I called on the radio. (All aircraft are given three letters for a call sign. Mine was GAX or (**G**olf) **A**lpha **X**-ray. Since all gliders are given the prefix 'Golf' we tend to drop the first Golf: Graham was GYZ or (**G**olf) **Y**ankee **Z**ulu).

'I'm struggling, Bernie, you had better make your own plans.' I could see him far below me losing out to the cold sinking air near the dam wall.

I had only once been above ten thousand feet so I cruised happily around the sky, contented yet keeping a sharp look-out out for other gliders. There were none. I had the stratosphere to myself, shared only by the odd Airbus on its way to Cape Town or Bloemfontein.

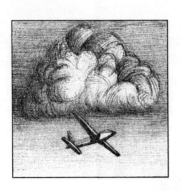

More threatening was the massive grey dome of cloud, now only a thousand feet above my head, inviting me into her bosom. Thirty seconds in that great sucker and I would be dead, having lost all orientation. I wasn't instrument rated, nor was my glider and, in any event, cloud-flying in gliders is strictly forbidden in South Africa. The canopy of my glider began to shudder alarmingly in the powerful lift so I hurriedly left the thermal and its dangerous cloud-top, deciding this was the day to investigate the meandering oxbows of the Elephant River north of the dam. Could I reach Liddletown? I had never flown that far from the airfield and it suddenly dawned on me that this could be the day for my first true cross-country flight. A street of clouds beckoned, seductively, fifteen kilometres to the west.

Turning your back on the airfield for the first time and flying out into the great unknown is one of the momentous highlights of soaring, never forgotten. That decision is never taken lightly, the repercussions potentially fateful. My inner equilibrium disturbed as I travailed with the idea, I decided that an important radio-call was in order.

'Shafton Ground, this is Alpha X-ray,' I called the airfield.

'Go, Alpha X-ray,' came back the reply from the duty pilot of the day.

'Wind direction and strength, please.'

'Less than five knots from the west,' came back the reply.

'I'm at 11,000 feet and going for a walk-about in the direction of Nottingham Forest,' I called back. It was important to keep him informed in case of misadventure.

'Enjoy!' came back the reply. I could hear the envy in his voice and I pinched myself. Was this really happening? Was it just a dream?

In between the banks of clouds where the lift is found – every cloud marks the top of a thermal – are great troughs of cold sinking air. I glanced out to the west at the beautiful street of clouds at least 15 kilometres away. Could I make it? Flying into a gentle headwind would make the return flight easier and I made the critical decision: *Go!* Excitement and, in equal measure, fear teased me; I couldn't believe it was happening. Half way to the bank of clouds, having lost two thousand feet, to my relief I flew through another blue thermal. As I banked steeply to maximise the lift I found myself staring down the wing at Astonhouse where I had spent so many happy years teaching science. Nothing much had changed. Memories threatened to swirl around, taking the squash team on tour to Rhodesia, now Zimbabwe, happy hours spent coaching sport on the fields I could see far below me, but I quickly dismissed them. Flying is unforgiving for those who are unable to concentrate on the job at hand. I levelled the wings and set my sights on Nottingham Forest and the bank of clouds ahead. The thickly wooded terrain far below me looked distinctly unfriendly. I followed the old highway carefully: it's very easy to get lost on a cross country flight although Lake Msimang and the Tollroad further north, off my right wing, were still clearly visible. More sink disturbed me but I was still at 9,000 feet when I reached the bank of clouds with a sigh of relief and climbed all the way up to cloud base, now at 12,000 feet above sea level. *Oh, this was good. Life was good.* I was at least thirty kilometres from home and nearly three kilometres above the ground lying far below me.

A new voice came booming over the radio, chattering with another club glider, the unmistakable accent of a Yorkshire Dales sheep farmer who flew out of Pinnacles Gliding club. Pinnacles? Could I reach Pinnacles from here?

There are three tasks that are important milestones for every glider pilot. One of them was easy, *a 1,000 metre height gain* that every pilot would achieve within a few months of going solo. I had probably done that a hundred times, though none had been registered because nobody routinely carries a barograph. The *five hour endurance flight* was difficult enough but it was *the fifty kilometre cross-country flight* out of Shafton that had only been done a few times. The terrain and the conditions just weren't suitable. Pinnacles? Could I really reach Pinnacles? My stomach was turning, churned with equal measures of excitement and panic. Later, after my baptism, my friends told me how they had joked over the anxiety heard so clearly over the radio.

Yes, it was scary but, drinking so deeply from the cup of life, the forests far below held no terror.

'Whisky Echo, this is Alpha X-ray out of Shafton Gliding Club. I'm at Nottingham Forest at twelve thousand feet.'

'You're far from home, Alpha X-ray. What are your intentions?' I had met the Yorkshire man before, his voice unmistakable, the accent recognized world wide by lovers of cricket. *Geoff Boycott** is an icon.

'Tom, is that you, in Whisky Echo?'

'No, it's not… it's…' His radio signal was broken by static and I couldn't hear him clearly.

'Can I reach Pinnacles from here?' I asked.

'Yes…' More broken patter. Damn radios, just when I really needed to hear him clearly. I *was* panicky. Would the wise pilot turn and head back for the safety of the womb? Should I press on for my first 50 kilometre cross-country flight? More travail.

'What's the best route to Pinnacles, Tom?' I called again, not knowing that I had got his name completely wrong and was making an ass of myself over the airway for fifty kilometres or more, in every direction. There was nothing wrong with *my* radio.

'Fly towards… Mooi Plaas† and then go directly along the Toll road to Pinnacles.'

'You're very broken up, Tom. Which way to Mooi Plaas? Do I fly to the Toll road or do I fly via Swartberg?'

I *was* scared. In retrospect I was possibly even experiencing some oxygen debt at that altitude. Steadying my anxious mind and controlling my fear, I pondered a moment. Stupid questions, I would have to choose myself one of several routes. It was no earthly good, or heavenly either, asking him to recommend a route. I scanned the sky. Over

---

* The radio commentator who made the Yorkshire accent familiar to cricket lovers worldwide.
† Literally 'pretty farm'. (Afrikaans)

Swartberg I spotted a promising cloud. That was the way. In actual fact, it would have made no difference. With my height a straight glide would have taken me to all the way to Pinnacles but I didn't have the confidence to do that.

Shafton airport ground control was out of my range now but I could still hear the chatter from several of my friends' gliders in the air. I relayed my intention to fly on to Pinnacles and would they please prepare my trailer for a retrieve? 'Yankee Zulu, Alpha X-ray is at eleven thousand feet and pressing on to Swartberg and Pinnacles.' All I got from Graham was a buzzing on the radio. He was too low for me to hear his reply. I set my course for the nearest cloud and increased my speed to over 120kph for the sink that I knew I would enter, immediately I left the thermal. And so I did.

I could see the road meandering along towards *Mooi Plaas*, and a series of beautiful lakes to the west mirrored the harsh African the sun. I had never seen them from the air before, and now the Drakensberg was clearly visible to the west, silhouetted against the hazy sky. A swift glance took in the whole sweep from the magnificent Sentinel in the distant north, to Giants Castle and the Rhino in the south. That's all that my anxious mind would allow me to indulge in and I focused again on the task at hand. Swartberg was below me and surely the ugliest village in South Africa, ironically called Mooi Plaas, lay just ahead. With growing confidence I passed the Toll, free for me, and pressed on towards Pinnacles, now only 20 kilometres away. I could see the roofs glinting in the harsh late summer sun.

'Keep your speed up, Alpha X-ray, at least 100kph. By the way, it's Fred, not Tom. Where are you now?' Fred's radio was suddenly clearer. I heaved a sigh of relief, relieved at the encouragement from the vastly experienced pilot. Yes, I was going to make it.

'Thank you Whisky Echo, Fred... I'm at 9,000 feet with the Microwave towers on Piggott's Peak just off my left wing.'

'Can you see the runways, Alpha X-ray? They are straight ahead of you.'

I scanned the terrain ahead. Secretaries' Dam was clearly visible to the west of the town and there right ahead I could see the X of two runways clearly marked at the airfield, though they appeared tiny from my height, hardly recognizable. I was determined to make certain of the full 50 kilometres for my Silver C so I flew past the airfield and over the picturesque dam with its towering cliffs.

Below me I spotted Fred's Twin Astir as he waggled his wings. He had sighted me at almost the same moment. It was a relief and I turned back to the airfield, preparing to land on the unknown runway. I took a good look, announced my intentions on the radio and started to *sideslip* * with airbrakes fully open to lose height. I was climbing! What was happening? I realized that I had flown accidentally into another blue thermal; a new thought slipped uninvited into my mind. *Could I make it home again? Could I go through all that again, twice in one day?* I closed the airbrakes and concentrated on centring in the thermal. The variometer needle started banging on the top stop and, before long, the altimeter needle started winding its way steadily back to 11,000 feet asl. Never had I experienced such powerful thermic conditions.

'Whisky Echo, this is Alpha X-ray again. What are the chances of me flying back to Shafton?' I asked. 'I'm back at 11,000.'

'If you can make it back to Nottingham Forest, it'll be a cinch,' called Fred. I realized my flight would be downhill from the Forest, located on the edge of the escarpment, at about 6,500 feet, to Shafton which was at only 4,600 feet asl. Would the same street of clouds that had brought me unerringly to Pinnacles take me home? I looked south, searching for over-development of the clouds and worried

---

* A technique used to lose height quickly.

about the mist that would creep over the escarpment if the wind had, unbeknown to me, veered to the south.

'Shafton gliders, this is Alpha X-ray over Pinnacles at 11,000 feet. Is anyone receiving me?' I called home, more than fifty kilometres away, needing information.

A faint reply: 'Go, Alpha... this is... Uniform...' It was broken up but I recognized Andrew, our CFI's voice and the call sign of our double-seater. 'Wind direction at Shafton please, Uniform Bravo?' I loved the old double-seater training glider that Andrew was instructing from. It was the same glider that had taken me solo more than ten years ago. I could hear him calling the duty pilot at Shafton and he then relayed the information back to me. 'Still from the west, Alpha X-ray.'

'Thanks, Andrew. Alpha X-ray is going to attempt an *out and return*.' I said my farewells to Fred and the Pinnacles club and set my sights on the Toll road that would lead me home. The hot tarmac was still giving birth to bubbles of hot air, forming the same street of clouds that lay scattered along the highway. It wasn't long before I was again soaring high over Mooi Plaas, still the ugliest village in East Griqualand. Nothing had changed. I caught another boomer and then flew straight on to Nottingham Forest. The lakes on the Little Mooi had a strange foggy appearance that gave an illusion of smoke, with the clouds reflected in the water, and I pressed on with the wind now at my tail. Below, the whole vista of Shafton rapidly opened, with Lake Msimang the beacon that would guide me home. It was a straight glide, over the forests of indigenous Yellowwoods and exotic Pines that terrified us, stopping all foolish notions of attempting long cross-country flights out of Shafton. Being forced to land in a forest is often fatal. I slowed down in the lift when my variometer notified me that I was in rising air and increased my speed in the troughs of cold sinking air, arriving back at Shafton still 5,000 feet above the airfield.

'Welcome home, Alpha X-ray,' called my friend Carl, from his mobile radio. 'We've got the reception committee ready.' I could see the club bakkie parked where I would land. I opened my airbrakes and searched for some sinking air to circle in. The altimeter wound rapidly down and I prepared to do my circuit, concentrating on the task ahead. Most glider accidents happened on landing and launching and I was exhausted after the draining flight. *Concentrate, Bernie.* It was an uneventful landing, as I flew just a metre above the ground, losing speed until the glider stalled gently onto the soft grass runway.

As I opened the canopy the welcoming group of pilots surrounded my glider, helping me out from the cramped quarters as I loosened the parachute. Their solicitousness completely deceived me. *They're so nice*, I thought, as they helped me onto the back of the bakkie, with much back-slapping and hand-shaking. 'We'll put your glider away for you!' someone cried. What a fool, I was completely deceived by their smiles and guffaws, my tired mind not registering that we weren't driving to the clubhouse for the first celebration frosty but to the farm dam.

'Hey, what's happening?' Strong arms grabbed me and moments later I was swung high in the air, boots and all into the dam. I came up gasping for air, with Carl laughing in the water next to me and the rest of the crew cheering from the shore.

'That's the Afrikaner tradition,' he said, wiping some weed out of his hair, 'just in case you get too cocky!' It was only later that I discovered that an out and return to Pinnacles hadn't been done for 20 years, and then in a fibreglass ship with a glide ratio of over

1:40. It was an important lesson for me. Cockiness and over-confidence mostly is what kills glider pilots.

Next morning I woke late, a bear with a sore head, and it had nothing to do with too many frosties or baptisms in farm dams. I couldn't turn my neck to the left and looking upwards gave me sharp stabs of pain in the neck. All that craning of my neck, looking for other gliders and clouds, all the stress and anxiety was concentrated in a small joint at the base of my skull. I palpated the area, feeling the spasm in the tiny muscles that control the upper cervical spine movements and the fixated joint that was causing it all. Damn! Helen brought me a packet of frozen peas wrapped in a tea-cloth and I gingerly moved my head from side to side, knowing that a self-employed chiropractor needed something far more life-threatening than a stiff neck to keep him away from work. If I was a state employee, I would certainly have taken three days' sick leave, but there was no escaping the salt mines for me. Fortunately I knew that the best treatment for a *torticollis** was at hand. Scott would adjust the nasty subluxated joint that was giving me a throbbing headache and the stiff neck. Having said that, a really painful neck can be many times more painful than even the worst low back pain.

It took several weeks for me to return to planet Earth from Cloud Nine. Fortunately, just by closing my eyes I can, and still do, revisit that epic day whenever I choose.

---

* Stiff neck.

Chapter Sixteen

AN (IN)ADEQUATE EXAMINATION

The chiropractor should lose no opportunity to perfect his ability to make a correct diagnosis, not only from a point of view of the chiropractor, but from the stand point of the medical profession.

Dr John Howard,
Founder – National College of Chiropractic
Chicago (1910)

A limp is always an important sign to a chiropractor. It could, of course, be a sprained ankle, just a broken toe or an arthritic hip but it could also be a lot of other things.

No doubt about it, José was limping. I walked down the long corridor, watching his stride, he only a few paces in front of me, as we made our way to my consulting room. I thought of the neurologist who had lectured us so many years before: the examination starts with watching the patient's gait and listening to his voice: 'Good morning, Mr Ferreira.' What I really should have remembered was the old medical gag that he had used to introduce the lecture. That was the most important lesson he taught us that day, but I must have been half asleep or overslept and arrived late. That and the well-known trio of polys were at the heart of the lecture: polyuria, polydipsia and polyphagia.

'Good morning, doctor.' There was nothing wrong with his voice. The shake of the hand can give important information to the thinking chiropractor. Is there a tremor, are the fingers weak, is there wasting of the small 'intrinsic' muscles of the hand? Mr Ferreira's hand was normal as far as I could tell. Worry was written all over his face: he knew something was wrong so at least I knew that the cranial nerve associated with smiling and frowning was normal.

'What can I do for you, Mr Ferreira? What is your chief complaint?'

'My right leg feels weak.'

'Does your leg hurt?' I asked. 'Do you have pain in the back?'

'No, I have no pain.' That immediately had my ears pricking up. A weak leg with no pain? Unusual.

'Are you in good health, as far as you know? Any serious illnesses or trauma in the past?'

'Yes, I am in perfect health.' Mmm, I wondered.

'No weight change, is your blood pressure good?' I went on and on with the various questions that are an important part of the initial history that every doctor, be he medical, chiropractor and, I'm sure, dentist too would ask.

'No, I am well. All prima.' He had a slight Portuguese accent.

'When did you first notice the weakness?'

'About six months ago. I started having difficulty on the stairs. Then my wife noticed that I was beginning to limp.'

The quadriceps is a very important muscle in the leg. When it is weakened, most usually because of a condition in the low back, a limp becomes very noticeable.

'So what happened then?'

'My wife insisted that I go to my doctor. He couldn't find anything wrong, and referred me to you. He said I must have a pinched nerve in my back.'

I was thorough in my examination; at least, I thought I was, as I knew this was not a run of the mill case. I checked his hips, knees and ankles. I examined his back thoroughly. It appeared normal as far as I could tell with the tests at hand. An MRI might reveal something less obvious. All I could find was a weak and wasting quadriceps muscle in his thigh, the muscle that straightens the knee and, to a lesser extent, flexes the hip. Standing on the affected leg was difficult and squatting quite impossible; his knee immediately started to buckle under the weight of his body. Little wonder that stairs were difficult. I could find nothing else wrong with him and was puzzled. The x-rays of his back that he brought from his doctor were quite normal. However, I didn't ask one important question, and I didn't do one simple test.

I got a playful call a couple of days later from Jonathan Hyde, our local neurosurgeon in Shafton to whom I had referred Mr Ferreira. 'You didn't ask him if he could get it up, did you Bernie?'

Unseen by him I blushed: 'No, of course I didn't.'

'Well you should have, because he can't. I'll bet you didn't do a simple dip stick test on his urine either.'

'Nope,' I answered lamely. I had been thinking along the lines of Multiple Sclerosis or Muscular Dystrophy. Not for one moment did I think of a Diabetic Neuropathy. One simple question, and one simple test, that was all that was needed.

'Didn't any of your lecturers tell you that silly joke, Bernie? The one about the three students leaving the last lecture of the day.'

'I must have gone fishing that day, Jonathan. Tell me,' I said, hoping this time I might have an opportunity to offer an adequate repartee.

'Well, as I said, the three students were exhausted leaving their last lecture.'

'Yes, and then?'

'The engineering student thought to himself: *I am tired and thirsty; I must have coffee.*'

'Yes, and the lawyer, what did he think, Jonathan?'

'Don't interrupt, Bernie. I'll miss the punch line. The lawyer thought to himself: *I am tired and thirsty; I must have beer.*'

'That sounds better. Yes, our neurologist did tell us this yarn, but I can't remember what the last student said.

'The last student, Bernie, was a medic. He thought to himself: *I am tired and thirsty; I must have diabetes!*'

I was nearly caught out by Margaret Thompson too, because I had never seen a case of dysdiadochokinesia,[*] the longest word I know, but fortunately her mother came to my rescue. The Cerebellum is that part of the brain situated at the back of the head; it coordinates the body's movements, making sure that when you scratch your nose, your finger stops before you poke your own eye out, and that the cake fork doesn't do a tonsillectomy. Our neurologist had taught us two simple tests: with the eyes closed, rapidly touching the nose from about 25cm away and, the second, placing the hands on the lap and turning them rapidly over, back and forth in an alternating manner. I had probably done the test a couple thousand times, but never found anything unusual.

'Doctor, I have headaches,' said Mrs Thompson. There was nothing unusual in that. Most people get a headache now and again.

'Tell me about them. Everything.' I said, putting my pen down and focusing all my attention on my patient.

'They are severe, and I'm getting them everyday. If I wake up in the middle of the night I have a headache.'

'When did they start?'

She started being a little evasive, but it was only later, after the phone call, that I realized it. I also didn't notice that, from then on, she wouldn't look me in the eye when she was answering my questions. 'About a month ago. I fell and hit my head on a coffee table.'

'Hard enough to give yourself a little whiplash, do you think?' I nearly made the fatal error of forgetting to keep the proper order: Take the history, do the examination, do any

---

[*] Impaired ability to perform rapid alternating movements.

special tests that may be needed, and only then make a tentative diagnosis and a list of differential diagnoses (other possibilities). One of the great problems with specialization is that it tends to give doctors blinkers. To many a medical doctor, a blow to the head only means concussion and possibly more serious things like a burst blood vessel in the skull. Like boxers have. Of course, to some chiropractors a blow to the head may only mean an injury to the cervical spine. I thought for just a moment of several boxers I had treated over the years. X-rays of their necks showed severe degenerative changes of their spines. Repeated blows to the head can do terrible things to the head and the spine.

I had already started thinking along the lines of a subluxation in Margaret's neck which is the most common cause of headaches. That is why chiropractor's offices are full of headache patients. Research shows that about seventy per cent of headaches are *cervicogenic*, or coming from the neck.

The cranial nerve examination of Margaret's head was quite normal, and then came that boring test that I had done so many times. I gave a little yawn. 'Margaret, please lay your hands on your lap and rapidly turn them backwards and forwards.' I couldn't believe it: Margaret's right hand was hopelessly uncoordinated with the left. 'Do it again, please!'

Margaret looked at her right hand in horror. 'What's the matter with this hand? It won't behave.'

I prodded around the base of Margaret's head which was very tender, as were parts of her neck where she had indeed had a minor whiplash. The patient can have more than one injury, and more than one illness too.

'Please go and have these x-rays taken, Margaret, and I want to see you before you go home tonight.'

It was about half an hour after Margaret had left, that the phone call came through from a stranger. Margaret's mother. 'Sorry to bother you, doctor, but I'm Margaret Thompson's mother. Did she tell you?'

'Tell me what?'

There was a bit of a silence. 'Did she tell you how she got the injury?'

'Yes, she fell against a coffee table.' I was suddenly concerned about releasing private information to a total stranger over the phone.

There was another silence and I was beginning to wonder if the caller had hung up. 'I don't know whether I should be telling you this – please don't tell Margaret I phoned – but I am a retired nurse and I am worried. Her husband flung her against the wall.'

'Whew, really? Okay, I will keep it quiet. Thank you for letting me know. Goodbye.' I quickly phoned the rad lab and asked them to add a skull series of x-rays.

Margaret came back with her x-rays at the end of the day. She was subdued and miserable. 'I have a pounding head. I'm sorry but I feel awful.' Suddenly she retched and ran for the basin in the corner of my room. It wasn't pleasant.

After we had cleaned up the mess, I put up the x-rays on the box. The fracture of the base of her skull was quite clear, even to me. I don't look at skull x-rays that often and they can be difficult to interpret, but the crack went right through the cortex of the bone that makes up the base of the skull. This was no time to temporize. I picked up the phone, hoping that Jonathan Hyde's secretary was still at the office. 'Hello Jennifer, this is Doctor Preston, the chiropractor. Is Doctor Hyde perhaps still at the clinic? I have an urgent case.'

'He's at the hospital, doctor. If it's urgent just tell the patient to go straight to the hospital. What is the patient's name? I'll call him on his cell and let him know that someone is coming.'

I gave her a few details, hung up and then turned to Margaret. 'I'm afraid you have to go and see a neurosurgeon right now. He's at the hospital. First I must give him some details. Now…' I said, pausing and holding up the x-ray of her skull for effect. 'You didn't do that on a coffee table, did you?' Silently I thanked her mother for helping, even if it meant breaking certain codes of ethics. In my book mothers are allowed to do that but of course I never told Margaret. Laws of medical ethics are established to protect the patient. It was in that very spirit that her mum and I had conspired to break the law.

She was silent and looked down at her hands. I waited. Finally she looked up and said: 'My husband and I were having an argument. He had drunk too much again, and he took my arm and flung me against the wall. I hit my head very hard. She began to weep quietly and I passed her a few tissues, trying to remember the name of the famous man who reminded us that heavy hearts, like heavy clouds in the sky, are best relieved by the letting of a little water.

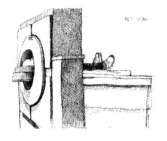

'Would you get dressed, please. I will drive you down to the hospital. I don't think you should drive.' The hospital was only a few minutes away and fortunately Dr Hyde hadn't left for home. I gave him a short history and my findings. He examined her with more sophisticated tests and immediately ordered an MRI scan. 'It's going to be a long evening,' he said. 'She almost certainly has a subdural hematoma, and the sooner we operate, the better are her chances.'

I went back to Margaret: 'You are going to be admitted, Margaret. Dr Hyde is just waiting for the scans. I'm afraid it is probably going to be an operation tonight. I will phone your husband and your mother if you'll give me their numbers.' I took a chance on her not asking how I even knew she had a mother. She just meekly gave me the numbers, still looking quite nauseous and green about the gills.

I phoned her husband first, telling him that his wife was in hospital; would he pack some clothes and personal belongings for her and get down to the hospital immediately. It was no time for incriminations. Then I called her mum. I didn't know her name so I just said: 'Good evening, this is Doctor Preston. Firstly, I want to thank you for having the courage to phone me – nobody knows, and nobody will know. You had better get down to the hospital as quickly as you can.'

Margaret survived the operation without any serious residual consequences. She left her husband at my recommendation, but a year later, I heard, she went back to him. I was unsure whether to admire her not. Women who take the 'better or for worse' that seriously reveal that they are indeed not the weaker sex. Or was she perpetuating the circle of violence? For me, husbands who beat their wives should be considered anathema to the association of men. They spawn a tragic world of sons who also are woman-beaters.

I hope Margaret's husband was suitably remorseful, for there was a price to be paid and it had nothing to do with money: about a month after Margaret's operation Jonathan Hyde had a fatal heart attack. He died in his prime.

For months I reflected on Margaret's case and wondered if her operation could not have waited until the next day. Was that one late night and a highly stressful operation the straw that broke his heart? Jonathan Hyde gave his all for his patients and it cost him his life.

It also came as what has become known as 'a wake-up call' for one Bernard Preston. If he didn't look after himself, then he wouldn't be able to look after his patients either. Jonathan Hyde was irreplaceable.

Chapter Seventeen

OF HIPS AND THINGS

I am standing upon the seashore; a ship at my side spreads her white sails to the morning breeze and starts for the blue ocean. She is an object of beauty and strength, and I stand and watch her until at length she hangs like a speck of white cloud just where the sea and sky come down to mingle with each other.

Then someone says, 'There! She's gone.'

Gone where? Gone from my sight – that is all. She is just as large in mast and hull and spar as she was when she left my side, and just as able to bear her load of living freight to the place of destination. Her diminished size is in me, not in her, and just at that moment when someone at my side says, 'There! She's gone,' there are other eyes watching her coming and other voices are ready to take up the glad shout, 'There she comes!'

And that is dying.

Turn Again to Life,
Mary Lee Hall

There are two pretty standard (so my friend Jeremy Thomas told me) orthopaedic answers to a married woman with an arthritic hip who asks the question: *When will I know it's time for the operation?* It's crude but for some reason it has stuck: *when opening your legs becomes too painful to have sex then you will know that it's time.* That, it seems, has become the yardstick, though I can't bring myself to use it. The other response is: *When you come here on hands and knees, pleading with me, then I'll operate.* Some doctors, of course, may have another response, thinking only of their next skiing trip. After all, every arthritic hip, young or old, advanced or otherwise is also, amongst other things, just a meal-ticket. For chiropractors, too.

But when Sister Margriet asked me the question, I didn't know how to answer: 'Mmm... well... I suppose... well, you will know, you know...' I stammered, thinking of Jeremy's first response, and going bright red in the face.

In my early days of encountering an arthritic hip, I wouldn't have taken on her case: 'You have an arthritic hip, Mrs Jones; there's nothing I can do to help you. I'm afraid you have to go and see Dr Thomas,' would have been my standard answer. But in Sister Margriet's case, Jeremy sent her back to me. 'She's just a little too young, Bernie. We can only guarantee these hips for about fifteen years. Do you think you can keep her going until she's sixty? It's only five years.'

I pulled out the x-rays and looked at them again. The right hip had advanced degenerative osteoarthritis. There was very little joint space and a huge amount of sclerotic change both in the roof of the hip (the acetabulum, as it is called) but also in the ball of the hip bone

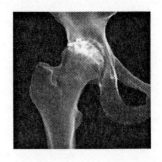

itself. Cystic changes in the bone confirmed that the bony structure was crumbling.

'I don't know, Sister Margriet. To be quite honest, I've never taken on a case like this, but let's give it a try. I can't charge you, but let's have 6–10 treatments over the next four weeks and see what happens.' I felt that was the least I could do to support a woman who had given up her all to follow her calling of poverty and chastity.

Whilst I was working on her I started thinking of the time a few years before when I had treated someone else for a condition that I thought was hopeless, and hadn't charged him, and gave a little snort.

'What's the matter? Don't you want to treat me?' She misinterpreted the sound.

'No, not at all. I was just thinking of a man I treated about five years ago and didn't charge...' I eyed my luxury 4x4 SUV parked just outside my window in the clinic parking lot.

'Want to tell me about it?'

'Make your next appointment just after lunch, and I'll tell you over a cup of coffee. It'll take a little time.'

'You know what, Bernie, this hip is feeling just a little better,' said Sister Margriet when she arrived for her cup of coffee, eyeing me as I munched on a cucumber and tomato sandwich.

'Really? You're not trying just to be nice to me?'

'No, not at all. Please will you go over those exercises again, though. I can't remember one of them. Now what about that man you were telling me about.'

'Hmff! That is an interesting story. He came to see me with advanced cancer of the sacrum, that's a bone in the pelvis...'

'Doc, I've got cancer, and I know I am going to die quite soon, but I am in dreadful pain. I can't sleep at night, and I am walking with a terrible limp. Nobody will touch me. They are all too scared they might hurt me. Don't people with cancer also have the right to treatment? Or do we have to go through the double agony of having a terminal illness, and being shunned by our friends who stop coming to see us, because they don't know what to say? Now all the doctors have added insult to illness, refusing to treat me except with awful painkillers that hardly help at all.'

'Well, it's true Mr Raaff, we do have to think of our reputations, and Chiropractic treatment could aggravate your condition, perhaps even seriously. Also the insurance wouldn't pay. Our whole training tells us to be careful not to treat people with cancer.'

'So I have to go through this treble agony! I feel as though life is spurning me. God has forgotten me, my friends are avoiding me and you doctors are refusing to treat me. It's a helluva lonely business getting cancer.'

'Yes, I can see that,' thinking how only the day before I had looked the other way when a man with no legs had passed me on the street in a wheelchair. I was afraid to catch his eye. What did disabled and sick people think when everybody ignored them because they were too embarrassed or afraid even to make eye contact?

'Will you at least examine me, and give me an opinion? I have money, I can pay.'

'It's not a matter of money, Mr Raaff. It's much more complicated than that. Today I will take a careful history and look at your scans, then if you will come back tomorrow, I will make extra time, and examine you, and then we will talk about it. Okay?'

His history was a sad business and I was glad he hadn't consulted me when the pain first started. The chances of me having made the correct diagnosis were relatively slim. As chiropractors we just don't have ready access to the batteries of blood tests and scans that are available to the medical world. Insurance companies will not pay for diagnostic tests ordered by chiropractors even in the very occasional, but essential, cases when we need them. Our hands are tied, and then if we miss an important diagnosis, they taunt us. In actual fact, Mr Raaff had consulted three different doctors, including a specialist, all of whom had missed his disease. It was in fact a sharp-eyed physiotherapist who had insisted on the bone-scan. The ensuing CT scan showed very clearly the area of increased bone density in the sacrum where the rapidly dividing cancer cells were proliferating. During my examination I was surprised how many of the orthopaedic tests for the sacro-iliac joint (SIJ) were positive. Was it the cancer that was effecting the SI joint, or did he just have an SI joint sprain? I had no idea, but it was most likely the cancer. Still, the condition presented very like a SI sprain. The dead giveaway was his gait. The way in which he walked was quite unusual, with a strange limp unlike anything I had ever seen. The disease was quite far advanced.

'What does the oncologist say, Mr Raaff?'

'Simply that it was diagnosed far too late and there is nothing he can do. I have apparently about five months to live. Five months of agony! Do you think you can help me? Will you at least try?'

All of my training told me to stay well away. There was only trouble awaiting me here. Maybe big trouble, but what did 'I care' think? Could I help, even if I did care? Was I prepared to try? Or would I just be robbing a desperate man?

'You write out a letter absolving me of all responsibility should anything go wrong, and get it witnessed by two people, and I will try for a month and see what I can do. For my part, I will do my very best. I will try hard not to make your condition worse, but you must understand there is a degree of risk. Just so there is no misunderstanding, there will be no charge.'

'You can't do that! I am not a poor man. You must charge me. The insurance will pay in any event.'

'Maybe, but I'm not at all sure I can do anything at all to help you. I am going against my better judgment, and I have never treated anyone with advanced cancer before. There will be no charge.'

During the first week I just did acupuncture on Mr Raaff putting needles into his buttock and down his leg. Not for the cancer, I wasn't treating the cancer, just his pain, and I used the points for a sacro-iliac sprain. Amazingly he felt just a little better.

'I'm sleeping better, Doc. Twice this week I haven't had to get up in the middle of the night and go through to the couch in the lounge.'

'You really think it's helping?' I didn't know whether to be pleased or not. Secretly I have a suspicion that my inner mind was hoping he wouldn't respond and that he would just go away! But no, Mr Raaff was a little better. So the second week I added a little stretching of the SI joint to supplement the needles. Then I had him doing home exercises and eventually began gentle mobilization of the joint. I wouldn't do a Chiropractic adjustment, but I used my *activator*,* surmising that increased movement in the hip would be beneficial and mobilization would be relatively safe. It was.

A week turned into a month, a month into three. I did everything I knew to help Mr Raaff's pain. It was draining, consultations took an hour, and we talked about life and death, the joys and the failures of his life. Never again did the subject of money come up, and some no doubt thought I was a fool, but my patient rallied, put on a little weight, and regained some of his colour.

'We can hope against hope, Mr Raaff, but don't be fooled. This is a good opportunity to put your life in order.'

He nodded and at the next consultation told me he had sold his business. I had no idea what he did – that was one area we hadn't discussed. Sometimes his wife would come with him, occasionally his daughter. I grew to know them well.

The end came very suddenly. He couldn't get out of bed one day, and went into a coma that night from which he never regained consciousness. Five days later he was dead. I wept briefly at that funeral, perhaps it was just the release of

---

* Device used by some chiropractors for adjusting the joints.

tension, not that I wanted him back with that continual gnawing pain. We had talked intimately of the love of God and I knew that he had just sailed out of sight. I was sure there would be a warm welcome awaiting him over the horizon.

I had the odd card from his wife, and his daughter became a patient, but then we all moved on and I put Mr Raaff away in some safe place of the memories.

It was some months later when my secretary put a call through one lunch time. 'Is that Doctor Preston?'

'Yes, it is I,' I replied in my bad grammar. Where did that come from?

'My name is Arbuckle. I am an attorney representing Mr Raaff's estate. Do you remember him?'

I drew in a sharp breath. *Please God, don't tell me I am being sued!* 'Yes,' I said nervously. 'How can I be of assistance?'

'We have some things we need to discuss, and I wondered if you could come to my office. I know you are a busy man – how would five thirty this evening, or next week, be?'

I cleared my throat doing some furious thinking. Should I contact my lawyer and take him with me? Should I get it over with as soon as possible? A quick look out at the printout of the afternoon schedule, confirmed that I could make it. 'Yes, I'll be there this afternoon, Mr Arbuckle. Where are your rooms?' We discussed a few details, and I had great difficulty focusing on my patients for the rest of the afternoon. Finally the hour came, and I left my clinic with a heavy heart, not knowing what to expect.

'Ah, Dr Preston. Please come in and take a seat. Can I offer you a cup of tea, or perhaps a whiskey?' This didn't sound like someone being sued.

'Er, no, I won't have anything thank you,' I answered anxiously. 'What is this about?'

The elderly man looked across the broad mahogany desk, meticulously tidy and said: 'You can relax. I have some good news for you.' He smiled. 'Mr Raaff, as you may or may not know, was a very wealthy man. About a month before he was diagnosed with cancer he ordered a luxury double-cab vehicle to be specially imported from overseas. It arrived in the Durban docks three weeks ago, and I am happy to tell you that, in his will, Mr Raaff specifically stated that you were to receive the vehicle. Now, isn't that splendid news?' He beamed, leaning back in his chair. I, for my part, was speechless.

'There's only one small problem. The VAT has to be paid, and that I'm afraid you are responsible for. It's quite a large amount of money, R52 000, in fact.'

I gasped. I work hard and make a comfortable living, but by the time I have paid the Receiver of Revenue, and my children's educational bills, and the cost of gliding and our annual holiday, there is very little left. Helen and I had few savings. The children knew that their inheritance was the best education that money could buy. Nothing more was guaranteed. Helen and I had scrimped and saved, jokingly telling the kids that once we reached sixty-five, we were going to go and *ski*: Spend (the) Kids' Inheritance.

My mother had died about a year before and left us a small amount, actually enough to cover the VAT with a little to spare, but we had decided to put it into paying off the mortgage on our house. 'Gosh, that's a lot of money to come up with so suddenly, Mr Arbuckle. Can I think about it?'

'Yes, certainly. You are under no obligation to accept the vehicle, but I'm afraid we can't sell it and give you the money. Will you let me know by the end of the week?' He told me the make of vehicle, and I gave another little gasp.

I sweated for the next few days. That inheritance paying off our death-pledge would put us out of debt for the first time, something we had been looking forward to for many years. 'You must take it, Bernie. It's a wonderful gift, and

I'm sure we can manage for another year with the bond. I can sell my old Beetle. That will bring something in,' Helen said.

'Yes, but...' I was being absurd. It was too good to be true. Was I being swindled? Something must be wrong. But what? I went and looked at the car in the showroom at Thompson motors. The salesman came around eagerly: 'Can I show you something? This 4x4 double cab, perhaps?'

'Well, actually, no... I don't want to buy it. But...' more stammering... 'could you perhaps show me the vehicle?'

He looked as confused as I felt but gave me the keys anyway. He was probably thinking: *Perhaps he will change his mind once he has test-driven it.* Why else was I there? The car was luxury beyond which I had ever dreamed of, way out of my bracket.

That afternoon I phoned Mr Arbuckle: 'We have decided to accept the vehicle, Mr Arbuckle. When do you need the money?'

'Mmm, there has been a small complication, Dr Preston.'

'Oh, if it's not to be...' I didn't know whether to be pleased or sorry. I still had a feeling I was about to see fifty thousand rand float away into somebody else's pocket. These sorts of things never happened in real life; there had to be a catch.

'No, the vehicle is waiting for you, but customs phoned me yesterday to say there has been an error. They were expecting the 2.8 turbo diesel, but the 3.2 Luxline has arrived. The VAT will be R62 000! Is that all right?'

I groaned. With something of a heavy heart, (was it heavy or was it elated? Was it confused, was it too good to be true?) I went back to the agent. The same young man came out effusively: 'I thought you might change your mind, sir. Would you like to drive it again?'

'Well, actually no, can I see the 3.2 Luxline, please?'

'The 3.2! Do you know how much that costs?' he said, looking at me doubtfully. 'Well, of course, if you want to test-drive it, I'll get the keys.' This time I didn't take it out for a drive. I didn't need to; it had all the bells and whistles. Now we could caravan in style! That turbo diesel was the tow vehicle of the year in the glossy upmarket section of the caravan magazine.

'That is a beautiful story, but there's no turbo diesel coming from me!' said Sister Margriet, looking out of my office window at the beautiful SUV.

'Yes, I know, but maybe there will be another surprise!' So we reviewed the exercises I had given her for her hip and also for her sacro-iliac joint and her back. Her limping gait had started affecting her back, and she was getting lumbago as well as hip pain. I reviewed my case notes, trying to recall a few specifics of what I had done. She had some very active trigger points in a muscle in the inner thigh that I had cross frictioned, a bit awkward with any woman, but particularly with a nun, but she was unconcerned, and I had placed a ring of acupuncture needles into points around the hip joint. Nothing unusual there. Then I had adjusted her hip joint and her sacro-iliac joint, all routine stuff. She was feeling a little better. I was rather surprised but could we get significant improvement and would it hold?

The surprise was that Sister Margriet's hip responded remarkably well to Chiropractic treatment, coupled with exercises and some acupuncture, the latter not used much after that first month of treatment. She comes in now for a monthly maintenance treatment – we both know I am not going to cure her – and she has stabilized at about seventy per cent less pain than she has suffered from for the last five years, and a great deal more mobility. She can now climb the stairs to where her office is located without much pain, something she hasn't been able to do for three years. Now that she has reached sixty, she is still putting off the operation. It will probably be necessary eventually, though, but we're holding thumbs.

Chapter Eighteen

A BEE UNDER THE MITRE

*We have, in fact, two kinds of morality side by side;
one which we preach but do not practise,
and another which we practice but seldom preach.*

Bertrand Russell

Even bishops, I discovered, can get angry. Very angry. When I went up for Communion I noted with concern the red face and the portly appearance. I had been trying to concentrate on 'He whom you should be focussing on' in church and, in fact, He was coming through loud and strong, only I wasn't

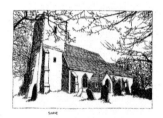

recognizing His voice. All I could see was a bishop with an angry face and a florid complexion. In my shallow spirituality I couldn't see the hand of God gesturing to me and saying: *Your next move could spell the difference between life and death for this man.* On the way out of church I briefly shook his hand and, on sudden impulse, then said to him: 'Bishop, would you mind pulling on my fingers?' He looked at me puzzled, but turned his hand over and we interlocked our fingers. As he pulled, I noted with horror as his thumb curled in towards his palm, a sure sign of an impending stroke.

I tried hard to dispel the disturbing and distracting thoughts but over tea they wouldn't leave. I spied Mary Ashton, the bishop's wife, on the other side of the room, chatting with a friend and made my way across towards her, cup in hand.

'Excuse me, Mrs Pritchard,' I said to her companion in tea. Turning to Mary, I said: 'I'm concerned about your husband. Do you think you could cajole Bishop Ashton to come to our home after church? It's important.' I passed her my business card with my address on it.

Oddly enough I had only met the bishop briefly, once or twice, in passing; oddly, as his wife Mary had been a patient for many years. They had recently retired to our little village of High Whytten, located in the hills above Shafton where I practised. Bishop Ashton took the occasional service. I had first treated Mary for a routine low back strain, the lot of young mothers, and then for headaches originating from the small joints and muscles at the base of her skull. The headaches had started after she had decided to go back to university and finish her Psychology degree and her neck didn't take kindly to the long hours of study. Actually it all went back to an injury in her childhood. *Children do bounce when they fall down the stairs, don't they?* Well, actually, no they don't.

I still vividly remember the day, more than fifteen years ago, when Mary came in for a consultation with the words: 'I've got a problem you can't fix.'

'Oh yes, and what's that?'

She eyed me with an unusual look on her face. I couldn't make up my mind whether she was close to tears or whether she was going to burst out laughing. They are, strangely enough, very similar emotions. 'I'm three months pregnant.' Now it was my turn. I also didn't know whether to laugh or to cry with her. Falling pregnant when you are forty-nine and the youngest of your three sons is sixteen is no laughing matter.

Over the years Mary had begun to treat me as her general medical guru, so I knew that she had not had a period for over three years. She had asked me, for example, about my opinion on *hormone replacement therapy*, generally in vogue in the medical community as routine for all post-menopausal women. I knew she had neither had a hysterectomy, nor an early menopause and, after a few routine questions, established that there was no family history of hip or spinal fracture. I also knew that both she and Bishop Ashton were part of a hiking group that took regular exercise, so we agreed on a bone density test and some Calcium Hydroxyapetite as a supplement. Personally, I am firmly against the carte blanche approach to HRT used by many doctors, having lost numerous female patients to breast and uterine cancer, and a few cases to stroke in their fifties that I suspected were HRT-related. There is indeed an increased rate of hemorrhagic stroke associated with HRT and the increased risk of cancer is well established. Obviously in certain extreme cases of menopause, and in women with a high risk of fracture there is merit.

An abortion was out of the question for them but I had strongly recommended an amniocentesis.

Mary firmly refused. 'I've heard it's a risky procedure and I'm not having an abortion anyway.'

'It's true, there is risk, but you really don't want to have a Down syndrome child, Mary.'

'You're trying to play at being God, Bernie. I suggest you let God be God, and you just be Bernie Preston.'

'Yes, but…'

She cut me off. 'No buts. Did you ever hear the old yarn, I know it's been discredited now, that there was once a woman who had eight children? Three were blind, two deaf and she was pregnant again. Her doctor diagnosed her as having syphilis.'

'So?'

'Well, the doctor recommended an abortion.'

'And?'

'She refused.'

'And the moral of the story?'

'Mrs van Beethoven named her baby son Ludwig.'

I sat, somewhat stunned. 'Sometimes, perhaps the exception proves the rule,' I finally said lamely.

So it was that little Martha duly arrived, two months after Mary's fiftieth birthday, a beautiful and perfectly normal child. I had managed Mary's back through the long and difficult pregnancy in the hot summer months in Shafton. She had frequent bouts of backache and acute pain along the *pubic rami*, her ankles had swelled and her blood pressure rose alarmingly at times. Mr Simmons, her gynaecologist, had been particularly incensed that she continued to consult me. He and I had angry words when I first arrived in Shafton,[*] an unregistered *ghostly* chiropractor and now, more than twenty years later, he still took an active dislike to both me and my profession, though we had never met.

'Do you think I should have a C-section?' Mary had asked me towards the end of her confinement.

'What does Mr Simmons say?' I had asked cautiously, not wanting to step on any corns.

'He is being insistent.'

'He's probably right, Mary. There has been some threat of pre-eclampsia.'

'Tell me again. What's that big word?'

'It's a condition of pregnancy in which the blood pressure rises dangerously, and there is protein in the urine. You are at risk, not having had a baby for over ten years and it could be a very difficult birth for both you and the baby.'

'Why don't you doctors use simple words we can understand? Yes, I know that, but the baby's position is quite fine and I feel ready for a normal birth.'

---

[*] Reference: *Frog in My Throat.*

'I'm afraid that's one decision I can't, and won't, make for you, Mary. You have to work that one out with Mr Simmons.'

'I'm down to have a C-section in two weeks. Is there anything you can do to help me go into labour?'

'Try hanging some curtains,' I said with a smile.

I have treated probably hundreds of women over the years during their pregnancies. It seems almost universally accepted that women must expect backache when they are with child, but I knew that mostly the backache of pregnancy was mechanical in nature rather than referred pain. It was related more to changes in posture and the release of a hormone called Relaxin, that allows for opening of the pelvic brim during birth, but making them vulnerable to sacro-iliac strain and pubic pain. I have yet to have a pregnant woman with backache who has not responded reasonably well to Chiropractic care. Most respond exceptionally well. Mary's baby was due in two weeks' time and ordinarily it wouldn't be a problem if she went into labour a few weeks early. Could I adjust her? Should I? An adjustment near term will sometimes start labour.

I had hesitated for a moment. In a younger woman I wouldn't have, but this was different. 'Mary, I think it's not wise. Mr Simmons is a specialist in handling births and I think it would be best if you listened to him.'

I still recall that Mary was not pleased with me but, like most women, she had her own way in the end. It was my secretary Sally who gave me the news. 'Did you hear, Bernie, that Mary Ashton had a daughter last night?' It was a full week before the scheduled C-section. It was over a month later that I saw a very contented Mary with her daughter in the parking lot after church one Sunday. 'Thank you for the flowers, Bernie.'

'It's a pleasure, Mary. Is all well?' I had asked.

'Everything is fine,' she beamed at me, 'except that lots of people think she is my grandchild.' She giggled like a schoolgirl. 'Callum is having a hard time amongst his friends who are quite sure he got some poor girl pregnant.'

I had laughed easily with her. 'And did God have his way with Martha's arrival, or was Mary proactive in some way?' I eyed her.

I had left church early to see an acute patient and Mary had taken her fussing baby outside. She looked around and then, in a conspiratorial manner, whispered in my ear. 'A friend told me that if a woman has an orgasm towards the end it will put her into labour. It worked but I'm not telling you how we managed it!'

I had burst out laughing, taking the proffered child and, looking down at her, thinking again of the miracle of birth. I had been at the birth of all three of my children but it never ceased to amaze me.

Now it was seventeen years later. I had met Bishop Ashton briefly at one of our Beekeepers' Association meetings several years earlier so I knew he kept a dozen or so hives to supplement his meagre stipend. Many Anglicans don't believe in tithing, or least our priests don't preach it very often, so the simile about the church mouse is not unwarranted. Those mice too, apparently had to make a vow of poverty, though they seemed to have ignored the chastity bit in our church. The extra income from the bishop's hives was what kept body and soul together and provided for not so little luxuries like sending their children to university. They didn't come to my office after that service but he did call a few days later.

'Is that Dr Preston? Mary asked me to phone you.'

'Good evening, Bishop.' He had phoned me at home. 'Thank you for calling. Look I'll get straight to the point. I was concerned at your appearance in church on Sunday, and I wondered if you would come in for a routine examination.

I'm a chiropractor, as you know, not a medical doctor, just so things are clear. There would be no charge, of course.' Touting for business, ambulance chasing and the like are frowned upon in South Africa, but for no charge I thought I could inveigle him into an examination.

Seventy per cent of the diagnosis is made from the History, and so it was in the bishop's case. The thumb sign, too, was important, of course. He had walked down to his apiary to check his hives, early on that Sunday morning before church only to find that they had been vandalised in the night. All fourteen colonies had been smashed beyond recognition, the boxes strewn down the path towards the forest. It was now unlikely they could afford to send Martha to university that year. Obviously he had got over the initial shock of finding his daughter's future in the balance but his blood pressure was still significantly raised. I was sure it had been very high that Sunday morning.

'Bishop Ashton, if you buy a dozen four-metre creosoted poles and get them planted in the ground around your apiary, I'll bring the wire and we'll erect an enclosure on a Saturday morning.'

'I've already considered that, Bernie. The wire is very expensive, I'm afraid.'

'Yes, I know, but once the heavy-duty spring cable that we use for launching our gliders becomes brittle and starts to break we just throw it away. It becomes dangerous actually and there are several rolls of the used cable stacked behind the hanger, still quite strong enough for your purposes. In fact it is high tensile steel, and quite difficult to cut.' We both knew that the scent of hives filled with honey was as strong as any pheromone. The thieves found it irresistible.

Early Saturday morning I took my two sons out to the Club and we loaded two rolls of used wire onto my trailer with the help of a couple of pilots who had arrived early to do the annual inspections on their aircraft. A kilometre of cable is very heavy.

We arrived at the Ashtons by eight. The bishop greeted us at the gate looking more relaxed. The apoplectic look had gone and I surmised that his blood pressure had dropped back towards a more normal value.

'Good morning, Bernie, the poles are in place. What have we here?' he asked looking into the trailer. I had encouraged him to call me Bernie, not long after we had met, years ago, but somehow the great man of faith would always remain Bishop Ashton to me.

The rolls of wire weighed over two hundred kilos each but the four of us managed to wheelbarrow them down to the remains of his apiary without too much difficulty. I had done plenty of fencing before so, by lunch, we had the three metre high fence in place, nicely tensioned with a puller not inappropriately nicknamed 'Satan' by my Zulu gardener. It crushed fingers if you weren't careful.

'You're going to need some more hives, Bishop,' I said, looking at the sorry state of what remained of his bees.

'Yes, and I had hoped to increase to thirty hives this season. Martha is going to university and I know we are going to need the extra income,' he said confidentially, out of earshot of the boys. I nodded.

During the next few days the bishop and his needs were not too far from the back of my mind. I kept thinking back to the days when I had first made a personal commitment to Christ. Sandy, my mentor, had insisted that the Lord had called the Church to go out and make disciples, not just converts, and there's a big difference. I was expected to attend a weekly discipling course. Tithing is amongst the many teachings of the Church and it was not omitted: *'Bring the full tithe ... and put me to the test, if I will not open the windows of heaven for you and pour down for you an overflowing blessing.'* I had already tested those windows and knew that it was no vain promise. They had helped me get through Chiropractic school. I decided to spend the next few months' tithes on the bishop and his needs. I ordered enough hive parts and frames to make up thirty empty beehives.

'Bishop Ashton, will you be home next Saturday morning? I have a few friends coming over to my place, and I wondered if you and Mary would like to join us.' In the meantime I had phoned several members of the parish whom I knew were handymen, and a couple of beekeepers who would not be averse to helping a bishop in need. Helen and Mary had arranged for a few of the wives to join us so the inner man was not to suffer.

Bishop Ashton's eyes were like saucers as we unloaded the dove-tailed hive parts and honey frames, all still unassembled. Others carried out half a cube of kiln-dried pine planks, still in the rough and the boys and I rolled out the 200 litre drum of wood preservative, an industrial wax. It wasn't long before the drum was up on blocks with a hot fire burning underneath it, and the workshop was abuzz with activity. The planers and saw benches were humming, hammers were busy and the boys and I were dipping the assembled hives into the boiling wax. The more experienced beekeepers were assembling the honey-frames whilst the carpenters were making up bottom-boards and lids for the hives. Discarded printer's sheets of aluminium completed the hive lids to keep adverse weather out.

'It's all very well having these wonderful hives,' the bishop said to me at lunch time as we were nearing the end of our task. We were all admiring the rows of neatly stacked hives, sandwiches and hot tea in hand. My sons were barbecuing couple dozen pork sausages over the hot coals. 'But how do I catch thirty swarms in a hurry?'

Just then one of the large commercial beekeepers ambled over to join us, hot dog in hand. He overheard the question. 'Very easy, Bishop,' he said pulling one of the finished hives off the stack. The swarming season is about to begin so all we need to do is to prepare the hives with a few used combs to attract the bees and then we put strips of bees-wax into the hive like this.' He demonstrated to the bishop how they did it in their apiaries. I too, listened avidly. 'I'll be putting out two thousand trap hives in the next month, so I'll just put yours out too. Some of those vandalised frames will do very nicely to attract the swarming bees.'

The African honey bee, *Apis mellifera scutellata* is one of the most dangerous animals on Earth, but she certainly knows how to collect honey. One of her characteristics is to swarm every year at the beginning of the honey flow, breeding new queens and spreading colonies far and wide. The specially prepared bee hives, hung up in trees a few metres above the ground, were exactly what the swarming colonies were looking for.

In two weeks the bishop had his thirty hives, filled with zealous bees all neatly secured in his apiary. Unfortunately, that is when his trouble really started.

Bishop Ashton had that apoplectic look again at the Communion rail. He singled me out after the service. 'The bastards cut the wire on Wednesday and stole ten hives,' he said angrily.

Mary invited us home for tea after church. 'Come on out. No matter that my husband will be a while tidying up after church.' Helen and I meandered out to their home taking Mary and Martha, now seventeen, to their smallholding. 'I'm very worried about Bishop Ashton. His blood pressure won't stand this stress,' I said to Mary and Martha.

I wandered down to the apiary while the ladies fixed up the tea things. Bushy old Azaleas protected their home from the bees and Bishop Ashton had planted rows of Bamboo around the apiary but that hadn't stopped the thieves. During the honey flow you could smell the sweet fragrance in the hives from several hundred metres away. The bishop had repaired the hole in the fence but the general mayhem was evident. The bees were angry and I had to duck behind some bushes so as not to get stung. I noticed a thin wire close to the ground attached to a strange looking contraption.

'Know what that is?' Bishop Ashton had walked quietly up behind me and caught me by surprise.

I turned swiftly round, momentarily fearful, like all South Africans caught by surprise, then, seeing him, relaxed. Turning back to the apiary I said: 'No, I don't know what it is. Tell me.'

The elderly bishop blushed. 'It's a man-trap.'

'A what?'

'Those trip-wires are connected to that device I made,' he said pointing to the gadget.

I stared, trying to fathom what it was. A fencing dropper had a short piece of galvanised pipe welded to it with a screw-on plug on one end. Later I saw the hole in the plug with a nail protruding and the twelve-bore cartridge in the pipe. Below the pipe was a mouse-trap, carefully placed so the heavy plate would spring up and strike the nail, just waiting for someone to fall over the trip-wire in the dark. No cheese in that trap, just a few dozen delicious honeycombs.

'Bishop! You can't do that. You might kill someone!'

He laughed. 'Come and I'll show you.' We were walking back up to the house when the ladies called us for ambrosial honey-tea and shortbread. On the way he took me through their lounge, opening the gun-safe to show me a beautiful pair of old Purdeys.

After tea, we strolled nonchalantly over to his workshop. Out of a cupboard he took a small box from which he pulled a faded orangey-red cartridge, very worn and tatty from years of use, passing it to me. I took the empty cartridge turning it over and over, catching a whiff of cordite, while he pulled out more small boxes.

'I was born on a farm,' he said. 'My dad gave me my first *four-ten** when I was nine. That's how I lost the end of this

---

* Small gauge shotgun.

finger. I was cleaning the gun and had forgotten to unload it,' he said, showing me his left hand. 'Then I got a twelve-bore on my fourteenth birthday.' All the while the elderly bishop was putting small amounts of a black powder into the cartridge with a small piece of wadding, and tamping it down. 'Won't be a moment,' he called, walking off briskly towards the kitchen bringing back, a few seconds later, a bottle filled with large white crystals.

'What's that?' I asked.

'This is Mary's coarse sea salt,' he said, with a grin, filling up the cartridge. 'That's what I used instead of the birdshot.' Then he fitted the cap and more wadding, crimping the shell and passed it to me. 'It won't kill but you can be certain that it will make for an awfully sore buttock.'

Twice in the next few weeks Bishop Ashton found the trap had been sprung but there was no sign of the thieves having been hit. His hives were still being molested though not devastated.

He came up to me after church a few Sundays later. 'I don't think we'll have any more trouble,' he said. 'The thieves were still messing my hives around so instead of salt I loaded the cartridge with buckshot.'

I put my hand to my mouth, obviously appalled. 'Don't look so anxious. I turned the shot ninety degrees away from the trip-wire and faced it into an empty paraffin can. I think the whole neighbourhood heard the shot go off at two in the morning and since then the hives have been untouched.' He was right on both counts. Almost every family within a radius of half a kilometre had heard, including the police, and the thieves never came back, although the arrival of the men in blue in the morning had the bishop scampering down to his apiary to dismantle the man-trap.

It was some months before I spoke to Bishop Ashton again. He was looking a younger, happier man and the raw fruit and salad diet that I had instructed Mary to start him on had worked wonders. An egg-and-bacon brunch was only allowed on Sundays. The honey flow from the Eucalyptus gum trees had been marginal but together with their savings, they had just managed to place Martha into the University.

'Bernie, I was brought up in the uMkhomazi River valley just downstream from the Josephine Bridge. When I was a boy I had a Zulu friend who took me bee-robbing sometimes and I remember that one Spring we had the most amazing amount of a pale yellow honey, quite unlike this from the Saligna gum tree,' he said, holding up a jar of the finely crystallised Eucalypt honey from our hives in High Whytten.

'I've seen it,' I replied. 'The plant is called uHlalwane.* It has small white flowers that produce copious amounts of nectar in spring. We joke about it at the Beekeepers' meetings and there is always an argument between the Creationists and the Evolutionists.'

'Why is that?'

'The lower lip of the flower looks just like the approach to the runway at an airport. It has a purplish nectar guide with a fishbone appearance, perfectly designed to direct the bee into the flower, and it even has a corrugated surface so she doesn't slip when she alights on the lip.'

'Hmm, interesting.'

'But there's a snag, Bishop,' I added, 'it only flowers every seven years or so. It's common name is *sewejaarbossie*.'†

'Yes, I know, but I was back in the uMkhomazi valley last weekend with the Bird Club. We like to go there because the high grassland is perfect Blue Swallow territory. I suppose it will always be home to me, the place I dream of, but this year it was very special, full of March butterflies and the grass was tall and beautiful.'

---

* Isoglossa eckloniana, known as buckweed, kiesieblaar, sewejaarbossie and hlalwane.

† Seven year bush. Prolific nectar producer.

'I'm afraid I wouldn't know a Blue Swallow from a Martin!'

'Not many do, but the difference is that the Blue Swallow is a threatened species. There are only about eighty nesting pairs left in South Africa. But to get back to my point, I met Sipho, my childhood friend again and I told him about my beehives. Sipho says this is going to be the year. He even showed me some of the plants.'

I looked at him uncertainly. 'It's more likely to be related to certain weather conditions than strictly every seven years.'

'That's true, but I have learnt that the Zulus out in the country often have an intuitive knowledge of the conditions. Would you help me take my hives out?'

The long and the short of it was that we took Bishop Ashton's hives, and ten of mine to fill the truck, out to his childhood home. Never in my whole life have I experienced a honey flow like that uHlalwane. Every ten days we took two supers of pale yellow honey off each hive. Six weeks later it turned off as suddenly as it had started. We had taken an incredible four tons of honey off the hives which grossed us an incredible R80,000 ($10,000) in under two months. It paid for the whole of Martha's three-year degree and I got more than double my tithe back. I thought back to Sandy's teaching all those years ago... *if I will not open the windows of heaven for you.*

A few weeks later, Bishop Ashton appeared in my appointment book. For no obvious reason he had developed a very stiff neck with pain radiating down his right arm. I decided it would be wise to x-ray him. Later, in the dark room, with the x-ray held up against the eerie red light, I pondered what I was looking at. The side of Bishop Ashton's head and neck was peppered with small round artefacts.

'Bishop, do you have any idea what these are?' I asked next day.

He came up to the x-ray box, looking mystified at the radiograph. Then he snapped his fingers. 'Ha, I know what that is. Sixty or so years ago Sipho and I were shooting *Kolgans* [geese]* and we had to cross the river to where they were feeding. He had my old four-ten and we crossed the river with the cartridges under our hats and only our head sticking out of the water, holding the shot-guns above our heads.'

I looked at him, intrigued.

'Sipho was about sixty yards off when his shotgun went off inadvertently. I was peppered with birdshot! Just as well it wasn't buckshot!'

I decided to photograph his x-rays with my digital camera – that was a picture to confuse my students at the Chiropractic College where I lectured one day a week. Fortunately the pinched nerve in his neck responded well to Chiropractic despite the huge arthritic spurs seen in most elderly folks' necks.

I wasn't surprised when a few weeks later I found Bishop Ashton had changed the lessons from those laid down in the lectionary. As soon as I saw them I knew what his sermon was going to be about.

---

* Spur Wing geese

Chapter Nineteen

IN WHICH AN HONORARY DAUGHTER MAKES HIS SUN PRAYERS

Thousands of tired, nerve-shaken, over-civilized people are beginning to find out that going to the mountains is going home; that wildness is a necessity; and that mountain parks and reservations are useful not only as fountains of timber and irrigating rivers, but as fountains of life.

John Muir, naturalist, explorer, and writer (1838–1914)

Unlike most, I had been looking forward to my fiftieth birthday for some weeks. It's not everybody who reaches fifty, and I had pondered on the fact that five of my graduating high school class never made it. Kevin was crushed against his car by a passing bus. Tom died in misery from dreaded leukaemia. Twins Jonathan and Jeremy were both killed, together with their girlfriends, on a drunken joyride barely out of school. And Samuel, our favourite, had a heart attack at forty-eight. It's a privilege to reach fifty.

I celebrated my half-century in style revisiting the mountains with my friend Sandy who had introduced me to his best friend[*] many years ago while we were still at university. Sandy and his family had emigrated some years previously, but he came back every year or two for a much needed holiday in his beloved Drakensberg Mountains. This year it coincided with my birthday. Helen of course, had objected but in the end she gave the trip her blessing, despite

---

[*] Reference: *Frog in My Throat.*

being excluded, knowing how much Sandy had contributed to my life.

Patients had found out about the big day and there were numerous cards littering my untidy desk. When Betty Button came in for her spinal adjustment she noticed, of course. 'Your birthday sometime soon?' she asked, tilting her head to the side in her inimical manner.

Betty was one of those elderly ladies with whom I had been something less than successful. A fanatical gardener, she had had numerous acute disc injuries in her early years and, when she first consulted me at seventy-four, I had been unable to help her debilitating sciatica. Her leg was lame and despite my best attempts nothing much had helped. Many years previously a medical colleague had popped my bubble: *'Do you really think that you should be able to fix every serious spinal condition? Do you think you're God or something? I refer patients to specialists every day. It doesn't mean that you've failed or anything. They just need treatment of a more specialized nature.'* Our Chiropractic history makes us feel like failures when we have to refer a patient to a medical specialist, fools that we are, with our fragile egos.

Unlike many patients who ended up in surgery, Betty had come back after her surgery for a monthly 'grease and spray', mostly just a gentle sacro-iliac adjustment and a mobilization of her very arthritic neck. Many surgeons are now advocating continued Chiropractic care after surgery. Adjusting her neck provoked extreme vertigo and I quickly concluded that it was not wise so I used my *activator* instead.

Betty and I had, for no particular reason, clicked from day one. Two years had passed since her first consultation, and although she was more than twenty years older than Helen and me, Betty became a firm friend. 'Do you hob-nob with your patients?' she asked one day. 'Will you come to dinner?' And so it was that we had dinners and bridge, picnics and concerts with Betty and her friends. Every consultation ended with a hug.

Life had brought Betty a lot of pain. Her husband had died early from a complication after a minor operation. Her two daughters had emigrated and one of them, Sue, had died in England of cancer. Every parent, I suppose, has a favourite; the trick is not to let the children know who it is. Sue had been the darling of Betty's heart. Her other daughter wouldn't talk to her because of some past hurt. Trivial or otherwise, it made no difference: to all intents and purposes, Betty was alone in the world.

'Yes, Betty, it's my birthday this weekend.'

'It's not on the 16th by any chance?'

'Well, actually it is. How did you know?'

There was a longish silence. 'Not your fiftieth? You weren't born in 1949 were you?' Betty was not an emotional person, a sweet smile, a hug but she just wasn't given to great displays of feeling. A tic started tugging at the corner of her eye, after she had posed her whimsical question, and her mouth twitched in an unusual way.

'Yes, Betty it is my fiftieth. My birthday was on the 16th August 1949. Why do you ask?'

Her face crumpled for the first time since she had consulted me two years before; that date was indelibly imprinted on her mind. She had named it 'Tears Tuesday'. It was a day of great rejoicing, and of much sadness. 'Sue was born on that day. She also died on the 16th of August, on her birthday. Your birthday, too,' she added. 'You are twins.'

'A good day to be born, Betty. A good day to die, too.' I sighed. Sue hadn't reached fifty either.

I really don't believe in the signs of the Zodiac and all that voodoo, but I had to wonder: was the fact that I was born on Sue's birthday the reason Betty and I had become so close? There certainly is something important in the firmament about birthdays, perhaps actually conception day. Just consider how many children are born on or about one or other parent's birthday?

And so it was that I became Betty's honorary daughter. It was a privilege.

'How are you going to celebrate your fiftieth, Bernie?'

'I'm not very popular with Helen, but I'm taking a hike this year in the mountains.'

'You are surprised you aren't popular?' she asked.

I shook my head, feeling not a little guilty. 'When I get back we are going to have a little celebration. Would you like to join us?'

'I'd love to.'

Those hikes in the Drakensberg with Sandy were definitely one of the highlights on my calendar. This was going to be the best of them all. I carefully packed a small bottle of my famous home-made honey mead, and Sandy always brought a half-jack of ginger brandy, wonderful on a cold mountain night sitting around a camp fire.

I woke that morning with a strange premonition: *you're going to see a snake, today.* In forty years of hiking I had never seen a snake in the mountains but, of course, all sensible hikers watch out for them: the famous Skaap-steker (a cobra) on the lower slopes and the very poisonous back-fanged Berg Adders high up in the colder regions, and always the possibility of stepping on a sleeping Puff Adder.

'Where do these strange thoughts come from, Sandy?' I asked after telling him about my dream. Sandy is a deeply spiritual man, and whenever I was in trouble I would email him for advice. He is one of those people who live close to God.

'I suppose it could just be something you read, or saw on television, but I would watch your ankles today, if I was you,' he smiled.

We had chosen to climb Mont-aux-Sources on that particular weekend. It is probably the most famous, and the most picturesque mountain in the Drakensberg chain, and source of two great South African rivers. As we drove closer

I grew increasingly excited. It was a whole year since I had been in the mountains and that weekend I would be turning fifty. The next day, in fact.

It was not long before our heavy rucksacks were readied, and we started like a pair of pack-mules for the base of the mountain, the peaks towering some 6,000 feet above our heads.

I could now write twenty pages about the beauty of creation as we wound our way up the mountain, through the sandstone layers with their weird shapes carved out by millennia of water and wind, and its caves, some of them big enough to house several families of the San people. We stopped periodically to 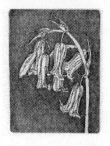 examine a tiny orchid, or peer at a kraal of the native people with their beehive huts; or Sandy would explain something about the famous rooigras (red grass). We kept a sharp lookout for Black Eagles, or a Lammergeier but all we saw were common kestrels and crows that twisted and turned in the cunning breezes that poured between the cliffs. There were fortunately no snakes but it is 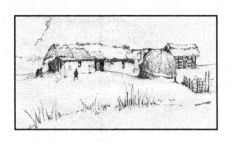 clouds that catch a glider pilot's eye; small puffy-white, innocuous looking cumulus that, within a few hours, grew into twisting, writhing, grey masses as we sweated up the mountain side. The first crack of lightning knocked the crop off a rocky crag no more than a hundred metres away. It had us diving flat on the ground and crawling towards a small overhang we had just seen. Anyone found standing on those slopes invited attention from those angry looking clouds.

An hour later, as the storm moved on, we continued our way along the path, now deep in water, our boots sodden, pressing on to the top of the mountain. There was no time to waste with the sun past its zenith and at least five hours of hiking ahead of us. I had long forgotten my premonition, but it was Sandy who gave a shout of 'run, run'! I had stepped right over the sleeping Puff-adder, ranked amongst the most venomous of Africa's snakes, waking him as I passed. Thick as my arm, it gave Sandy, walking close behind me, an angry warning hiss. He escaped death, saved only by a dream that caused him to keep a sharp lookout all day. I had forgotten all about the warning, never having heard of a Puff Adder lying in wait in a puddle of icy water.

We made the final climb up the chain ladders, and the last of the hike across the darkening African landscape. It wasn't long before we had our torches out, searching for the cave we knew was hidden on the side of the mountain. We had both slept there many times and it was not long before we found Crow's Nest cave, hungry and weary but inwardly invigorated by our encounter with nature in all its glory.

'Don't forget to wish me Happy Birthday tomorrow, Sandy,' were my last words that night.

'Of course not, I even have a small gift somewhere here,' he said gesturing towards his pack.

My fiftieth birthday dawned as magnificent as any morn can. The storm had washed the dust from the air, there was not a cloud in the sky and the early morning temperature was around five degrees. I was woken by the early morning light cascading into the cave, and lay quietly doing my back exercises. I was stiff from the long climb and the hard rock on which we had slept, softened only by a thin foam mattress. Turning every hour in the night and even sleeping on my tum, breaking a cardinal Chiropractic law, was inevitable. Another friend, Peter, had introduced me to a set of exercises called the Sun prayers, done to a series of nine grunts, in worship of the Sun, I suppose. I was very hesitant because of my conservative background, but I particularly liked the exercises although I could never bring myself to chant the Hindu mantra. The stretching of the muscles of the spine, the arching of the low back and the contraction of all the muscles in the body, starting with the toes and going right up to the neck and face, done in a slow rhythm to the chant of the numbers 1–9 had become one of my daily routines. The coordination of rhythmical exercise to a specific deep breathing programme, together with the chant, was a discipline that required considerable focus of body and mind.

Sandy woke and quietly watched me for some time stretching and counting. I became aware of his watchful presence and clambered over to his corner of the cave, pouring him a cup of early morning tea.

'Those are interesting exercises,' he said. 'Where did you learn them?'

I squirmed, not sure that I should tell him. I felt not a little guilty doing my 'Sun prayers'. Eventually the truth came out. Sandy said nothing, but was obviously doing some thinking. It was he who had so many years before taught me the value of starting the day with God. He had brought a tiny pocket-size New Testament with him, and so it was that we sat on the edge of our cave, great steaming mugs of tea in hand, with the mountain peaks around us, and the province of KwaZulu Natal spread out far below.

It is here that two of South Africa's great rivers rise. From Mont-aux-Sources, towering just behind our cave, a trickle bubbles out of the ground, winding its way westward, collecting other rivulets, forming the mighty Orange River, now known as the Gariep, as Africa seeks to delete all signs of its colonial heritage. The river meanders across Southern Africa eventually finding its way into the Atlantic Ocean, thousands of kilometres away, having cut through mountains and deserts, gorging out diamondiferous pipes along the way and watering the homes and farms of millions of Southern Africans. Here too, is the source of the Tugela River, starting with a spectacular 3,000 foot drop over the basalt rock face, no more than a few hundred metres in front of our cave, the second highest waterfall in the world. Like its sister, both sourcing from the 'Mont', the Tugela supplies the nation on the eastern seaboard, winding its way ultimately into the Indian Ocean. The Sentinel ahead demanded cameras, along with the Tooth, and its Tooth Pick, peaks that Sandy had climbed in his crazy mountaineering days. To the south and east the panorama of KwaZulu Natal spread out, all seen from almost twelve thousand feet above sea level. It never fails to impress and we sat quietly, silenced by the magnificence of Creation. Finally Sandy picked up his Bible: 'Would you like to read with me from the book of Galations?' he asked. 'I have chapter 5 to study today.'

'And these are the fruit of the Holy Spirit, signs that will characterize those who follow after the Christ: Love, Joy, Peace, Patience, Kindness, Gentleness, Faithfulness, Goodness and Self-control,' Sandy read. He stopped and I wondered why. Normally he would read the whole passage and then we would dissect it.

'How many chants did you say you had to do? Was it nine?' I saw him counting, and he looked up with a smile. 'There's the answer to your dilemma. Dedicate those exercises to the other Son, the Son of God who created the Sun, and chant those nine words every day, and I daresay you will have the most powerful mantra of all times.' So it is that I still do my Sun Prayers, chanting the nine fruits of the Holy Spirit that should characterize the life of the Christian. I say *should* because it is taking me a lifetime of being shaped by God into the kind of person who is ready to spend eternity with Him. Starting with the word *Love* and ending with the very un-hip word *Self-control* it has become, and continues to be one of the most sobering, life-giving challenges to start each day. Do the words have mystical powers? No, I don't think so, but I cannot say that mantra glibly.

We clambered about the mountain tops, hiking south to the famous Pinnacles, swam in the crystal clear pools and shared the difficulties and joys of our lives. Finally the day ended, still with hardly a cloud in the sky, we finished what was left of the mead and brandy, and next morning sadly found ourselves hiking back to reality. We lunched in a river bed, soothing our tired feet in the water, a mountain Bottle Brush, as beautiful as any part of creation, its deep red flowers vivid even to my colour-blind eyes clung to the edge of the ravine just a few metres away. I was putting some honey onto a Provita biscuit when another reality hit me: 'Sandy, you forgot to wish me Happy Birthday yesterday.' We both roared with laughter before Sandy reached into his pack, pulling out a small parcel, obviously a book. It was a short history of the San people who once lived in those mountains, exterminated by Zulu and European alike.

No one could have wished for a finer fiftieth birthday.

Chapter Twenty

GREAT-UNCLE ETHELBERT

Life is short. Be swift to love! Make haste to be kind!

Henri Frederic Amiel

The two ends of a circle seem to meet with relative ease. Drive around a traffic circle and you'll know what I mean, but the ends of an ellipse seem to have to wander through the unknown, like comets, waiting for half a century or more before they find each other again.

The two ends of my ellipse found each other one weekend, eighty-six years after they started off on their long journey, about the same length of time, give or take ten years, that it takes Halley's Comet to revisit our solar system. It happened this way:

The Chief Flying Instructor of Shafton Gliding Club phoned me one Tuesday evening: 'Bernie, we are giving the children from Ethelbert Home a flip and lunch this Saturday. Could you come and spend a few hours on the winch, please? I'm afraid there will be no flying for members.'

'Ethelbert? That's an unusual name, Andrew.'

'Yes, it's an orphanage near Durban; quite a progressive place.'

'Ethelbert Children's Home? It rings a bell. What a splendid idea – that will make their day.'

'Sadly, for a few it will be the highlight of their year. Some people just dump their children and never come back, or not for ten years.'

'Count me in, Andrew. I'll be there.'

Saturday dawned bright and sunny. Soon pristine white cumulo-nimbus clouds, with grey underbellies, began to bring promise of strong updraughts and heavy downpours. Pilots arrived early at the airfield behind Lake Msimang, dragging out the gliders and doing their daily inspections, and then schlepping them to the launch point before the children arrived. Others went off for some party fare and it wasn't long before the bus from Ethelbert Children's Home in Malvern near Durban arrived, crowded with children eagerly looking forward to a day in the sky. They stared at the powerful winch that would soon be towing them high into the heavenlies, gathering around the gliders and gazing wide-eyed at the instrument panels. With their seventeen metre wingspans the monster gliders were impressive, lying in wait for their pilots and passengers. The children watched intrigued as the two 1,200 metre long cables were dragged from the heavy drums on the winch, out of sight over the hill. Some were anxious, all were excited, clamouring to be first into the sky. Fortunately there was plenty of lift that day and it wasn't long before the gliders were thermalling up under the clouds. A few stomachs turned green as the gliders turned in tight circles to stay in their thermals, but the children's faces remained enthralled and excited.

What's the connection between comets in ellipses and gliders in their circles? you may well ask. The answer is a story of tragedy, but not despair, of death for one small boy but life for thousands of children, all born out of the faith of one couple, and carried on by generations of hard-working visionaries.

'Hello,' I said to the man who was obviously in charge, when he came to the winch with a few of the children to watch. 'Please keep well clear because sometimes the cable can break and it may be dangerous.' We had never had a serious injury at the club but I hadn't forgotten what a cable had once done to my own glider.[*] I certainly didn't want this to be the first time something ugly happened to a visitor at the club. That cable was lethal under tension.

'It's good of you chaps to do this for the children. My name is Tom Corbishley.'

'Hello Tom, my name is Bernie. Bernard Preston, actually. Do you work at the Home?'

'No, actually, I don't, but my great-grandparents started Ethelbert Home nearly a hundred years ago, so I try to spend one day a month doing something interesting with the children.'

The radio crackled, interrupting our conversation. Two gliders were loaded and ready for take off. I shoed the children well clear of the winch, and the launches were routine. Both gliders found thermals within a few minutes, and climbed their majestic way up to cloud base. Watching gliders never ceases to excite me and defying that great force of the Universe, gravity, is an unending source of satisfaction. The visitors too were enthralled, chattering excitedly while waiting their turns. We all stood with heads upturned, watching as the gliders were sucked up by the warm air rising under one of the clouds.

One of the girls, no more than ten, sidled up to me now that it was safe, and took my hand. 'Can you fly those gliders too?' she asked.

I recognized a small girl longing for attention. I looked over at Tom and raised my eyebrow. He gave a silent nod, so I climbed back into the cab of the winch, lifting the child onto my lap, and giving her a hug. She nestled in my arms and I realized how vulnerable these children are. 'Yes, I fly here most weekends,' I replied. I couldn't help noticing her tatty clothes and shoes, obviously hand-me-downs and far too big.

'Will you be my pilot then?' she asked innocently.

---

[*] Reference: *Frog in My Throat.*

I laughed. 'We could ask the boss. His name is Andrew. Perhaps, Mr Corbishley will talk to them over lunch. What's your name?'

'Sarah,' she said shyly.

'You can call me Bernie, okay Sarah?' Everybody is on a first-name basis in gliding. There are no formalities, even with children.

I turned to Tom. 'My grandmother was a Corbishley, and I vaguely remember mention of Ethelbert Home. Do you think we could be related?'

'I suppose we could,' he said, a little doubtfully. Preston seemed very far removed from Corbishley. 'What was her name?'

I scratched my head thinking of my grandmother, long dead. 'We called her Nana. Let me think, what was her real name? She died about thirty years ago. I would guess she was born late in the nineteenth century.' The small bakkie arrived to tow out the cables, interrupting our conversation and my train of thought. Sarah grumbled when I had to get down from the winch to hook up the cables. She crawled right back into the crook of my arm after I climbed back into the winch cab.

'I think her real name was May, Tom. Does that ring a bell?'

'No! You're kidding me, Bernie! That's astonishing. Ethelbert had a sister called May. Your Nana may have been Ethelbert's sister. That makes us second cousins! My grandfather, Harry, was May and Ethelbert's older brother.'

I pushed Sarah over to the corner of the cab. She gave another squawk and I gave her little hand a squeeze before climbing down from the cab and going over to Tom. We shook hands rather awkwardly, and I thought to myself: *to hell with this* – and gave my new-found cousin a very firm embrace. Tom was a little embarrassed but we chiropractors are unashamedly touchy-feely people. In the good sense, of course.

Thomas and Frances Corbishley were married in England in 1876 and emigrated to the province of Natal in South Africa some two years later. Thomas established the law firm of Corbishley, White and Co. in Durban and proceeded to have a large family, whose descendants still live all over KwaZulu Natal. Tragedy struck when my grandmother, Frances May Corbishley, was six – her younger brother Ethelbert, aged only two, drowned in four inches of water in a storm-water drain outside the kitchen door.

Being a couple of great faith, Thomas and Frances decided to donate the money that they would have spent rearing Ethelbert to start a home for orphans, which was duly established in 1907. Ethelbert Home still stands today as a tribute to the faith of a young couple who tragically lost their son, and the flame is still carried on, ensuring that the Corbishley dream dies. Ethelbert Home is a progressive institution with sixty children, having been the first in South Africa to introduce the concept of orphan children living in their own home with foster parents.

Sarah got her flight with Uncle Bernard, and when the goodbyes came, she looked up at me and said, in the innocence of childhood: 'Uncle Bernie, can I go home with you?' Tom tried to shoo her away. 'Just wait, Tom,' I said. I got down on one knee, like I advise all my patients with low back conditions to do when they need to bend. 'I'm afraid not, Sarah, but can I come and visit you?'

She looked at me scornfully. 'Everybody says that, but nobody ever keeps their promises.' She tugged away and ran off to their bus, deep raking sobs shaking her little body. I was left, still on one knee, not knowing what to think. Would I be another of the many who had deceived this gentle little girl with their lies?

I shook Tom's hand more formally, as we bade farewell. 'Well done, Tom,' I said. 'I'm impressed by the way you

help keep the family flame burning. We shall meet again.'
We swapped email addresses.

When important things are happening in the ether they often seem to become intertwined, not letting us escape from the essence of what is happening. A patient, Harold Ellis, approached me during the treatment of a nasty sciatica: 'Doc, would you sponsor me for the Comrades Marathon, if I am able to run? We are trying to raise money this year for a children's home.'

'Which home?' I asked. It was a stupid question. I already knew the answer.

'It's a small place near Durban. You won't have heard of it – it's called Ethelbert Home.'

I didn't enlighten him but his eyes did open wide when he saw the figure I committed myself to. Now I had to fix him so he could run. Runners become quite neurotic during the last few weeks before marathons. They have invested upwards of a thousand hours in training but a dose of flu, a sprained ankle or painful sciatica can blow it all. At ninety plus kilometres, one of the most gruelling ultra-marathon races in the world, the Comrades is very unforgiving of athletes who try to run with an injury or illness.

I made another deal with Harold. 'I will give you this course of treatment for free, Harold. If I get you well enough to run, will you donate the whole amount to Ethelbert Home? If I don't, then I will donate the cost of the treatment to the Home.'

He looked at me with a grin: 'You're on.'

'There is only one condition. You must do exactly as I say in the next four weeks. Even then, there is a fair chance you won't run.'

Sciatica is a nasty condition for a runner. The pinched nerve passing down the back of the thigh hinders one from swinging the affected leg forwards, making it impossible to run and can even make walking difficult. There is a simple test that will usually confirm if the pain in your leg is coming from your back:

Sit on a normal chair and ask someone to raise your non-painful leg parallel to the ground. Note what you feel in your good leg. Now drop the good leg and ask your helper to raise the leg that hurts – if there is pain in the leg and you can't straighten it, or if the pull is much stronger than the other leg then you more than likely have sciatica. If, with your leg raised, flexing your head onto your chest makes the pain worse then you are in trouble. Do something quickly.

'Harold, you must go to bed for three days, but do these exercises every half an hour. Every hour get up for as long as you can manage, but not more than an hour. You are not to sit at all, nor bend and, if the weather is warm enough, then get into the swimming pool for ten or fifteen minutes. Lie on your back and kick and, in the shallow end, run gently on the spot. Please ask your wife to bring you in for daily treatments – remember you may not sit – so you must lie on the back seat of the car.'

Harold ran the Comrades and achieved a good time, all things considered. It cost me my donation plus the cost of twelve lost consultations but, as I would have given the Taxman forty per cent anyway, it didn't hurt quite so much. Harold paid his share very happily.

The Sunspots kept disturbing the ether above my head. Ten days before the Comrades a Chiropractic student from the College phoned me: 'Doc, could you help out at our Chiropractic tent on Comrades day?' Their usual consultant was on holiday, and they couldn't treat the athletes without a qualified chiropractor in attendance. It was a long drive from East Griqualand but I felt that I had something extra invested in the Comrades that year.

'Yes, certainly. When must I be there and where is the Chiropractic tent?'

'It's in Malvern, Doc. Just up the road from a children's home.'

'Ah,' I said, pausing for a moment, guilt ridden. I had completely forgotten little Sarah, but it seemed as though I was not going to be allowed to forget her. 'It wouldn't be Ethelbert Home would it?' I asked.

'Yes, how did you know?'

'When you have a spare hour then I will tell you, but meantime just assume I know where it is.'

That evening I pulled out my gliding logbook where I had jotted down Tom Corbishley's email address. *Tom, I am coming to help out at the Comrades Marathon this year and will be in the Malvern area. Is there any chance Helen and I could take Sarah out for the weekend?*

My ellipse was complete and the story of Sarah I will have to leave for another book. Suffice it to say that the Preston holidays thereafter required a cottage for six and we regularly started making weekend trips to Durban.

Chapter Twenty-One

SURGERY

First, do no harm.

Hippocrates

Thought I'd write and let everyone know why they haven't heard from Marjorie.

She had another back surgery in January in which the doctor said her spine was almost totally closed off. She was put in a body cast which also went down the legs. About one week later she was in a lot of pain. Had some scans done and found out it didn't hold. So, she went for another surgery. Two weeks later I took her to Emergency as she had awful pain in her legs. They took x-rays and scans and said everything looks fine, gave her a pain shot and sent us home. That was Sunday. Monday when I visited her, her back was soaking wet along with her bedding plus a temperature of 40 degrees Celsius. So back we went only to find out she had Staph infection all the way to the spine, in the blood and in the bone. She was in the hospital for two weeks very, very sick! She is now home as of Monday. For now she is equipped with a wound vac that is in her back, draining the infection, that gets taken out and cleaned out every two days. Also she has an I.V. in her arm with antibiotics. So this is why no-one has heard from them and Tom doesn't use the computer. That's the latest of what's going on with us.

Sonia.

Private correspondence.

215

Most of the world has a terror of back surgery and, perhaps, rightly so. However, I believe in good surgery when the indications are right. One of the reasons I so respected Dr Jonathan Hyde's work was that he almost never operated on sore backs, but only when the pain radiated down the leg and he certainly wouldn't do lumbar surgery for something as spurious as headaches. I had numerous patients whom, after struggling unsuccessfully with pills, and physiotherapy or Chiropractic, lead relatively normal lives after his ministrations. Of course, there were others not at all satisfied but, considering that he only took over when everybody else had given up, I reckoned his results were pretty good. But after Jonathan died, things changed...

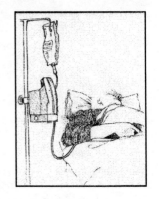

Some people do seem to get a raw deal out of their bodies. Perhaps one should blame life. Was it her genetic profile that gave issue to Mrs Marjorie Sampson's poor health? Or the fall down the stairs when she was only three, fracturing two important little pieces of bone in her lower back? Perhaps it was the car accident when she was eighteen and she wasn't wearing her safety belt, or was it the creeping mid-life obesity? Perhaps it was all four, plus a few others; like a lifetime spent at an office desk with little passion for sport or exercise. No doubt about it, Mrs Sampson had one of the nastiest frames I knew. A new patient, in my early days in Chiropractic, her neck was a struggle for me. Surprisingly, her lower back, where the fractures had occurred, gave little trouble. In medical jargon we call it a 'stable spondylolysthesis'.

Clearly Marjorie had let herself go to seed. It's difficult not to make value judgments in the health business. The fact of the matter is that lifestyle has a profound effect on health and Mrs Sampson's was shocking. So was her case record; the gamut of trauma, advanced arthritis and medicine abuse had all taken their toll. Still, it was surprising that she had so little low back pain.

'Doctor, do you think you can help this awful neck of mine? I get blinding headaches,' she finished, rubbing her neck and shoulders. Her right arm hung limply at her side, obviously withered. She supported it protectively with her left hand.

'When did they start, Mrs Sampson? Can you remember?'

'Oh, years ago, I can't really remember.'

'Ten, twenty, thirty years ago? Did you have headaches when you were at school, for example, or when you were newly married?'

'No, not at school, but I do remember having them when the children were small. They made me miserable, even back then, for a couple of days almost every week. Now hardly a day goes by when I don't have a headache,' she said, craning her neck, and rubbing her shoulder with the hand of her good arm.

'Any trauma, bad falls, car accidents?' It was a rhetorical question. Any observant person could easily see she had been injured, but I needed the details.

'Yes, I was in quite a bad car accident when I was twenty. My cousin was driving, and went through a traffic light on orange when he really should have stopped.'

'Did you hit another car?'

She nodded. 'We hit a car that turned in front of us, and my head went through the windscreen. The glass cut the nerves to my arm,' she said, gesturing to her partly paralyzed right arm.

'Which way were you facing when the cars collided?'

'I was talking to my cousin. Sideways.'

'So you didn't see the car ahead? You had no time to tense the muscles in your neck? A safety belt?'

She shook her head. I was asking too many questions. I presumed she was negating all three.

Fortunately for Marjorie she could still use her hand and wrist and a clever surgeon had rerouted a muscle which gave her some use of her shoulder. Still it was obviously very disabling as often occurs in so-called OOP or 'out of position' road trauma. Mrs Sampson was facing her cousin, her head turned to the side. Later, during the examination, I saw where the glass had ripped through the *brachial plexus** in her neck, severing many of the nerves to her arm; a safety belt would have saved her from much of the painful course that her life ultimately took. Research has now been done proving that a safety belt reduces the incidence of moderate-to-critical injuries by fifty per cent.

In major trauma one is never really sure which demon will haunt the patient. Was it the terrible injury to her cervical spine caused by the whiplash, as she sat chatting to her cousin, oblivious of the impending crash? Or was it the blow that her head took against the glass, shattering the windscreen and causing a serious concussion? Was it the rupture of the nerves to her arm or the psychological disadvantage of being partly paralysed? Or, perhaps the headaches and painkillers that blighted the rest of her life? Or, like multiple exam questions, was it *all of the above*? Brought into the emergency rooms with a ruptured artery and severed nerves in her neck, she had come very close to bleeding to death. It was, all in all, a miracle that she survived the accident.

'Are you otherwise in good health? Any other problems?'

She didn't say anything for a few moments, gathering herself, and then going on. I could see she was a strong woman, not the kind that would readily burst into tears. She

---

* Important large group of nerves leaving the neck and travelling under the collar bone and through the armpit to the arm.

had come to terms with her disability, knowing how lucky she was to be alive, thanks only to the paramedics who arrived on the scene within minutes, and some very skilled surgeons. Nothing in those days could have been done to save the nerves to her right arm. 'Yes, I have lost one kidney. The doctors tell me it is from all the pills I take for these headaches, and the other kidney isn't working well. They say I will be on dialysis before too long.' She looked steadily at me without a sign of emotion. She had taken over twenty analgesics per week for many years. 'I have some backache sometimes, here down the bottom,' she added, gesturing, 'but that's not too bad. It worries a little, occasionally.'

'Are the headaches constant? Do they throb? Where are they located?'

'It feels like a tight band around my head. No, it doesn't throb. Just a dull, constant pain, often here over my eye or sometimes here at the base of my skull.' She pointed to the upper part of her neck, where the spine meets the skull.

'Do you get nauseous, or are you overly sensitive to light or sound?'

'Not really. I just have horrible headaches, week after week; they have ruined my life.'

I was not unduly concerned about the so-called *traction or inflammatory* headaches* (they would have killed her years ago). There was a distinct possibility that *psychogenic* headaches were an aggravating factor. A moderate degree of depression was inevitable but in my assessment was not the cause per se. *Cluster* headaches† were also an unlikely possibility that I should consider.

---

* *Traction and inflammatory headaches* are usually of sudden and severe onset and may be accompanied by memory loss, confusion, changes in speech or vision, or loss of strength in or numbness or tingling in arms or legs or fever and a stiff neck.

† *Cluster headaches* are usually severe, unilateral and are typically located at the temple and around the eye. They are usually brief, lasting from a few moments to less than an hour. They occur in clusters in a period of a few weeks, usually not returning for months.

'Do these headaches occur at the same time every day? Can you set your watch by them?'

She shook her head. 'No, not at all. They are often bad when I wake up, or when I go to bed. In fact, I can get them at any time of the day, and they often last all day.'

'And your low back? Does that trouble you? Do your legs ever ache?'

'I get a little pain down there sometimes but really it's nothing.'

I nodded, starting with the ranges of motion of her lumbar spine.

I made an interesting discovery that day. During the examination of her lower back, instead of sitting in the normal way on my treatment table with her legs down and feet on the floor, Marjorie Sampson misunderstood me and put her feet on the foot-rest of the table, so that her knees and hips were slightly flexed. The old fracture and subsequent slippage in her lower back were undeniably visible in a way that the ordinary examination might often miss. I reckon now that I can spot nine out of ten *spondylos*, as we call them, during the physical examination.

'My blood pressure is well controlled with medication.' Fortunately she wasn't also a smoker. I could see that she didn't have the wrinkled facial skin that, continuously starved of oxygen, gives smokers away no matter how advanced their moisturising creams are.

I looked at the thick wad of x-rays that she had brought in, giving a little shudder. It would probably take me an hour just to look at them. 'When were the most recent taken?' I asked.

'I haven't had any for at least five years.'

I glanced at the envelopes. 'This is fantastic, they go right back to your original accident!' I opened the first set of thirty years old grey plates, eager to see what they showed, putting them up on the viewing box. Long minutes passed while I gazed, perplexed. Certainly there were signs of injury, but nothing that might predict the severe degenerative changes seen in the most recent radiographs. On that first set of x-rays there were very mild compressions of two Cervical vertebrae, loss of the normal curve which could have been due to muscle spasm but was more likely due to tearing of ligaments, and the fracture of one *uncinate process*[*] that would certainly cause quite serious problems in the future.

The rest of the radiographs recorded the progressive onset of osteoarthritis over the years, rampant towards the end, as the fixated joints, starved of nutrients degenerated. Subluxations of the joints cause stiffness, reducing the free flow of oxygen and vital substances to the joints, and causing toxic waste products to accumulate in the fixated joints.

After the examination, which revealed a very limited range of motion in the lower neck, but fairly normal in the upper neck, and really very little difficulty in the lower back, I took her through to the x-ray room and took new radiographs of her neck and lower back. Not in my short career, nor since, have I seen such a shocking lower neck. At four levels there was almost no disc space, and the degenerative changes in all the lower joints of her neck were those of a ninety year old. The upper neck was largely spared as was her lower back.

'Was your neck very stiff after the accident?'

Silence. She didn't answer.

'Mrs Sampson, was your neck stiff after the accident?' I repeated.

She lifted her head. 'I could barely move my head for three months after the accident. I wasn't allowed to drive, not because of my arm but because I couldn't turn my head to look out of the side windows.'

---

[*] Tiny piece of bone in the neck that protects the nerve from a slipped disc. When fractured in trauma, if not carefully managed at the time, it leads frequently to severe arm pain in the future. Often not detected.

The effects of trauma to the neck, such as Marjorie Sampson had experienced, are two-fold. Firstly, there is the initial accident, which could cause varying degrees of damage. Relatively minor fractures of the vertebral bodies are common and occasionally more serious fractures of other bony parts; then there are the injuries to the soft tissues: the discs, ligaments and fascia, muscles and nerves. Nothing could change that, the damage was done. But the second effect, in the long run usually more serious, is very treatable but is often completely neglected by modern medicine. I thought of some recent research done at my Alma Mata in which it had been clearly demonstrated how induced fixations in the spines of white rats would cause degenerative osteoarthritis to start in less than twelve hours. Subluxations result in reduced movement in the spine, reducing nutrient flow to, and waste products from the tissues, and the resultant progressive degenerative change, now scientifically proven to be caused by fixations, is often worse than the original injury. I had never seen such a mess. Mrs Sampson was only fifty years old. What was to be done, if anything?

'I'm afraid you and I are between the proverbial devil and the deep blue sea, Mrs Sampson. If I do treat your neck, there is considerable risk of making things worse. If I don't, then if the headaches don't ruin your life completely, the pain killers certainly will. Do they actually reduce the pain?'

'I think they help a little, but as much as anything, I just have a need to do *something*. I have to try and help myself.' She had aged prematurely, a weary look about her, her hair almost completely grey, and the lines and creases around her eyes deepened as she gave me her first little smile. Suffering, pain and too many pills had left their mark. All because a young man never stopped at a traffic light, and because she didn't know that prevention of the progressive arthritis had been available. No one had told her.

'Are you willing to try? I have been everywhere else except a chiropractor. They told me my neck was far too bad for manipulation. It would be dangerous.'

'Maybe *they* are right,' I said with a smile. 'In the lower part of your neck anyway but fortunately the upper neck is largely spared and that's where I think your headaches are coming from. There are also a lot of trigger points that we can treat, though other therapists have no doubt worked on them over the years – did physiotherapy not help?'

'Yes, it brought relief for a day or two, but that's all.'

'Mrs Sampson, I need at least an hour to go through all these x-rays. A complete record like this is quite valuable both to you and various clinicians, by the way. Don't ever throw them away, or lose them. I am going to give you some exercises and gentle stretches of the muscles today, and then we will start the treatment proper tomorrow. Please bring your husband with you, so that we can discuss whether you really want to go through with this. As with all health care there is risk,' I added. I spent the next hour carefully analyzing the radiographs, and photographing them with my digital camera. A series like that, tracing the progressive deterioration, was invaluable.

The following day we thoroughly discussed the possible treatments.

'Just how safe are these Chiropractic adjustments, Dr Preston?' Mr Sampson hadn't been in favour of his wife consulting me.

'That's a very legitimate question, Mr Sampson. The relative danger of manipulating the lower neck is considerable. There is near *ankylosis** in that part of the neck. It has turned to concrete but there are possibilities of mobilizations and different degrees of manipulations that we chiropractors use. There is less danger, and I would in any event expect better results from adjusting the upper neck and

---

* Severe stiffness or, more often, fusion of a joint.

upper back. The overall prognosis, I'm afraid, remains bleak.'

'What about her lower back where you say she has had some fractures?' He looked doubtful.

'Your wife has very little pain or disability in the lower back, Mr Sampson, and I personally think it best to let sleeping dogs lie. She also has quite advanced arthritis under the knee cap from a condition known as Patella Alta.' I explained the good prognosis in her knees with Chiropractic treatment. She was not really obese, nor had she had any knee injuries, so there was no advanced arthritis in the knees proper.

Analgesic-induced headache was also something to be considered but, for the moment, I decided to leave that on the back burner. There were so many strong indications that her headaches originated in her neck. I doubted that her headaches were actually caused by the analgesics that she was taking to relieve them. There was no doubt whatsoever though that the painkillers were a huge debilitating factor in her health, and could have been actually aggravating the headaches they were supposed to be relieving.

The results of my treatment of Mrs Sampson's headaches were more or less as expected. Her headaches were reduced by about half, in both severity and frequency – provided she came for a consultation every two or three weeks. Not really satisfactory, but she was satisfied initially. We managed to get her analgesics consumption down to less than ten a week, but she still had dreadful headaches periodically. Her knees also responded remarkably well to my standard treatment for knee-cap pain. I never touched her low back. Nothing warranted it, in my opinion. A simple set of exercises was all she needed. Other chiropractors might disagree and some surgeons, too.

Several years later, I was stationary at a traffic light on my large *dream-machine*,[*] and watched a car go sailing through on red. Fortunately no one started off early, and I had a sudden thought: *I haven't seen Mrs Sampson for a year or more. I wonder how she is?* It was one of those inexplicable flashes generally known in the profession as 'going fishing', and of course Mrs Sampson phoned later that day to make an appointment. She limped in with a stick looking seventy.

'Nice to see you, Mrs Sampson. I had a déjà vu moment this morning when I saw a car go through a traffic light, and it made me think of you. You haven't had a consultation for some time – nearly three years,' I finished, checking the file.

She looked at me, and then dropped her head. 'I made a mistake. No, two mistakes.' She wouldn't lift her head and look at me in the eyes. I noticed her hair was thin and unkempt, and she was beginning to look frail. Her face had taken on a grey, even haggard look, and I felt sorry for this woman who had suffered so much. I waited.

Finally she went on. 'I got tired of your maintenance treatments, and my doctor urged me to go to a specialist, to see if more couldn't be done. The surgeon said the headaches were caused by the fractures in my lower back, and that I must have a back operation.'

'A back operation!' I exclaimed.

'I don't know why I didn't accept that the help you were giving me was all I was ever going to get. He bullied me into having the operation.'

'But you weren't having much pain in your back, were you?'

'No, but he said the operation would help my headaches.'

I just shook my head, now angry, at a doctor who would so mislead a desperate woman. 'Did it help your headaches?'

'No, it didn't help at all, and after the operation I had a terrible time with my back. I got an infection, and was in and

---

[*] Reference: *Frog in my Throat.*

225

out of hospital for weeks, and then had to have a second operation.'

'Oh, no! Your neck?'

'I had a terribly sore neck for a month after the operations. Now I have a sore back *and* headaches. Actually my headaches have been much worse.' She began to sniff, the first show of emotion during all our consultations. I passed her a tissue.

My eyes dropped to her bare knees where I noted with horror the large angry red scar associated with a total knee replacement. Her lower right leg jutted out alarmingly in what we call a valgus deviation. 'And your knee?'

'After the back operation I started getting terrible sweats and high temperatures; I was in an out of hospital for the next six weeks. They said I had a Staph infection and I had to have a drain fitted. Then I started getting pain in my legs. First they thought it was coming from my back, and so I had another operation. Then they said it came from my arthritic knee, and I had to have a knee operation. That was two months ago.' She was drifting a little, not realizing she was repeating herself.

During the examination, I became more and more angry. The knee replacement was a total botch with her lower leg jutting out at an acute angle. No wonder she now needed a stick. The pre-surgical alignment was within the normal limits, as were the femoral-tibial joint spaces. Most of the arthritis had been under the knee cap, not in the knee proper. All ranges of motion in the lower back were now painful and limited, especially forward flexion, and the stiffness in her neck had worsened. I didn't know what to say – nothing could undo the medical mismanagement and negligence that I witnessed.

I felt very weary, effete, almost unable to go on, wishing that I had explained the benefits of Chiropractic in a more convincing way and with more authority. I would make a very poor second-hand car salesman.

Chapter Twenty-Two

NECKS, KNEES AND GRIEFS

Is Chiropractic safe? The answer is yes. Only 1.5 serious adverse events per million manipulations occur. This is safer than many conventional therapies for the same problems. Is it completely safe? The answer is no. Adverse effects do occur and well-developed guidelines exist that should be followed to minimize the risks.

Wayne B. Jonas, MD,
Director, National Institutes of Health, USA.

If you are tall and heavily built, then your knees may become a problem when you are old and grey. If you are seriously overweight, then your knees are likely to cause you pain. If you've had leg injuries, usually from sports or trauma, then your knees may inhibit your mobility. If all three are true, and particularly if you are of the female sex... then unfortunately you can expect hell from your knees.

Mrs van de Merwe was a big lady but her knees weren't the reason for her consultations. She was one of the first patients that I inherited after my senior lady partner retired. I grew very fond of the woman but she gave me nightmares in that first week. A local doctor's wife, she had come to my colleague for treatment for unremitting dizziness that responded to only one thing – a Chiropractic adjustment.

She was my first patient one Monday morning when I had just returned from our annual congress. The courses had been on the relative danger of manipulation; in fact, the possibility of a causing a stroke. A Chiropractic nightmare, though extremely rare, the subject had been fully aired and discussed. A new examination procedure called Wallenburg's test that might be useful in predicting a high risk patient, though it was unproven, was demonstrated and in a hands-on session we had work-shopped the test repeatedly on fellow colleagues.

I arrived back in my office not too concerned about *stroking* a patient, as it was called, but more aware. The chairman of our Chiropractic Board (and he should know; his office was specifically formed to handle such occurrences) informed me that he was aware of only two cases of stroke after Chiropractic manipulation in South Africa, though there may well have been more. In the eighty years of our history nearly a thousand chiropractors must have each given of the order of 300,000 neck manipulations. That makes adjustments of the neck one of the safest medical procedures, certainly much safer than the 'minor' vasectomy that came very close to causing my own demise. Nobody had warned me either that vasectomies also come with a significantly increased risk of prostate cancer.

As fate would have it, Mrs van der Merwe had a severe attack of vertigo while we were all away at congress and was not at all pleased that Shafton had been without a chiropractor.

'How can you all possibly go away for four whole days and leave us without a chiropractor?' she demanded. 'That is highly irresponsible of you as a profession. I think I am going to report the whole lot of you to the Board,' she finished, with a twinkle in her eye.

'I wish you would,' I said with a laugh. 'It's the Board that requires us to go each year to congress and, if we don't go, then we stand to lose our licences. Continuing education is the buzz word these days.'

'Do you learn new things?'

'Yes, new things but of course we also need refreshers on old stuff that one just doesn't use all the time.'

'Like what?'

'Other causes of headaches, for example, and common diseases that one might forget to consider in making a diagnosis. Then there is always a course on radiology, and this year we had a lecture by a neurologist on stroke.'

Mrs van der Merwe nodded.

'You are right though, it does make things difficult for our patients if there is an emergency. Now, what's the problem?' I had never treated her before.

'I have had dreadful dizziness for the last four days, and my husband's pills don't do a thing. The world is spinning.'

I examined her carefully and was disturbed to see that Wallenburg's test was wildly positive. Not only did she get dizzy, but she had a severe attack of *nystagmus*,[*] during the test. I was apprehensive, partly I confess because she was a medical doctor's wife. It would have made a compelling headline for an eager young reporter at the *East Griqualand Herald*: CHIROPRACTOR 'STROKES' DOCTOR'S WIFE.

I considered my warning carefully. 'Mrs van der Merwe, I am afraid you fall into a higher risk category, so I am going to mobilize your neck for three days. That will probably fix your dizziness. It may take a little longer, but it's a lot safer.

She looked at me dubiously. 'Will it be different to the treatment that I am accustomed to from your colleague?'

I nodded and proceeded with my conservative treatment. But my mobilization didn't help and, at the fourth consultation, she was angry. 'Why did Dr Thompson have to retire? She wasn't that old, and you youngsters don't have the same grit as the older chiropractors. Just get on and give me the adjustment I need.' I should have been pleased.

I weighed up the pros and cons. The chief pro was that her neck had been adjusted at least twenty times over the years for dizziness. The treatment had been successful, and she hadn't had a stroke. Plus it is middle-aged folk who, mostly, are at risk; Mrs van der Merwe was in her seventies. That

---

[*] Involuntary movements of the eyes.

was before Wallenburg's test came to the fore, though, and I had no way of telling if it had only just become positive. Perhaps it had been positive all along, but my colleague would never have heard of Dr Wallenburg and his test.

Anyway, I adjusted Mrs van der Merwe's *atlas*[*] only once. It fixed her vertigo and she didn't have a stroke. One of the gurus of Chiropractic, a man called Palmer once said: *Find the subluxations, fix it, and then leave it alone.* So I adjusted her atlas, and then left well alone! But as she left, I said: 'Mrs van der Merwe, why don't you let me have a look at your knees?' I could see there was a problem from the way she walked and the difficulty she had standing up from a chair.

She gave me a steely look on her way out the door. 'Do you think you can help my knees? I am due to have two knee replacements in five weeks' time. I'm dreading it.'

'I won't know until I've looked. Come in next week and bring your x-rays.' I knew the surgeon would have ordered plates.

Mrs van der Merwe was a big lady, nearly six feet tall. On top of that she was very heavy, 117 kilograms. She had been an ace hockey player in her time, taking many knocks on her knees, and of course she was female; the dice were loaded against her. I was not surprised at the osteoarthritis that became clearly evident as my examination proceeded; the grinding in her knees was horrific, but interestingly much of the pain came from under her kneecaps.

Kneecaps were something I learnt very little about when I was studying Chiropractic. I knew their anatomy and function, of course, and that the undersurface degenerates in a condition called *Chondromalacia Patella*. A Chiropractic lecturer, perhaps biased, informed us that surgeons like to remove them and that was about it.

---

[*] Top bone in the neck.

'And Clarke's test was positive.'

'Er, Clarke's test, er… what's that again?'

'You know, for Chondromalacia Patellae.'

'Oh, yes, of course,' I lied.

The Principal of the new Chiropractic College had invited me to be part of the Internship programme when the clinic opened. I had hesitated, knowing that academia had never been my forte. 'You'll learn quickly, don't worry,' he said, and so it was that the blind found himself leading the sometimes not-so-blind. As soon as the intern left the Clinician's office I quickly pulled out McGee's text book of Orthopaedics and started to read up on Clarke's test. It was a very simple test for C.P. and for the next week, I did the test on every patient who came into my office in Shafton.

'Doc, why are you testing my knee, it's my neck that hurts?'

'I've learnt a new test, so I'm examining every person this week for degeneration of the cartilage under the kneecap, so that I get to know what normal feels like.' The first patient I experimented on gave a cry of pain. The test was excruciatingly painful and I was reminded, as with all orthopaedic testing, how important the artful examination is. These tests were designed to put pressure on, or stretch certain tissues of the body and, carelessly done, they can quite seriously aggravate the condition.

'Is Clarke's test still positive?' I asked the intern the following week when he brought me his case notes for a signature.

He looked at me a little incredulously. 'I'm sorry, but I thought you had no idea what Clarke's test was. Do you use it regularly in your clinic?'

'I've done Clarke's test on well over two hundred knees, young man. Don't be so impertinent.' I didn't tell him that I had examined all those knees in the last week. Or that, as of one week ago, I had never heard of the test. 'Make sure you do it very gently and carefully. That test can be excruciatingly painful,' I added, knowledgeably.

'Yes, I've discovered that already.' He looked at me with a little more respect.

'How's the treatment going? Hmm, I see the patient has fifty per cent less pain. That's impressive. Now, how are you treating the patient? Ah yes, that's good,' I said, digesting all that he was doing. 'Can I suggest you add some quad setting exercises?'

'Gee, Doc, you really do know about patellae. Our lecturer said most of his notes were hot out of the research, and nobody who had graduated more than two years before us would know anything about it.'

'Ah, poppycock. Much of this stuff is very basic and there's nothing new about quad setting. Actually, I like to do it with the heel fixed to the floor and the knee fully extended so the patella slides easily up and down in its groove.' I didn't tell him that I also had access to the internet and its amazing how much you can learn in a week when you don't want to sit and look like a fool. The now partially-sighted clinician was just one step ahead of his intern. That week every patient, no matter what they came to the clinic for, had their patellae assessed and, if found wanting, treated. I was surprised how often Clarke's test was positive and how quickly patients responded to the treatment which, like the test, could be quite painful if not gently done. After only three treatments one elderly man said that his knee, which had been painful for five years, had improved remarkably. 'I didn't know that you were so clued up about knees, Doc. I should have asked you years ago to treat my knee.' In fact, it was I who should have known that he had the problem.

'And you know what, Mr Penter? Your back is also a lot better this week because you're not limping so badly.' I had told him previously that I would need to see him at least once or twice a month for the rest of his life because his arthritic gait was affecting his back so badly, but it was only his kneecap that was making him limp. The young intern's treatment programme was working admirably.

The following week I treated at least forty knees with chondromalacia patella, some admittedly in its very early stages, and I was several leagues ahead of the intern. 'Do you think ultra-sound might help?' I asked him.

He looked a little dubious. 'You know, one of our students is doing research on ultra-sound and he found it to be very ineffective.'

'Mm, that's interesting,' thinking how once I had used a dud ultra-sound machine for a whole year without knowing it wasn't functioning.* 'Maybe I will leave it out of my treatment regimen. I do find Chondroitin Sulphate helps a little.' He raised his eyebrow, and a little smile pursed his lips. I could see him thinking: *So the ol' fart knows a little more that we give him credit for!* In those early years at the College clinic the old fart was on a very sharp learning curve.

But back to Mrs van de Merwe: She was big boned and heavy, and she had very arthritic knees. Painful knees. After about two weeks of treatment, her husband came in with her. 'Ah, Doctor van de Merwe, it's good to meet you at last,' I said.

'Yes, I've come in to see what you are doing for my wife's knees. You know, she has less pain, and she's walking better. I'm curious to see how you are treating her.' He had been retired for about two years but that didn't stop his wonderfully active and alert mind. Retirement gave him time to get involved in helping establish clinics for AIDS patients. He had a strange voice, not an accent, not nasal... just odd. I couldn't place it.

I examined her knees again. Clarke's test was now nearly negative, but the grinding from within her knees was just as bad as ever. Flexion was still very limited. 'I will now start

---

* Reference: *Frog in my Throat.*

seeing what I can do about your inner knee, Mrs van de Merwe,' I said, 'but that is going to be far more difficult. What really concerns me, is that we may simply be delaying the knee replacements by six months or a year.'

'Is there any point in starting then?' she asked in a quick rejoinder.

'That depends on how much you want to avoid surgery. Remember it's not one major operation, it's two.'

'I don't want the ops at all!' she exclaimed. 'My best friend died two days after a double knee operation. 'From a complication in the lungs,' she added.

Her husband nodded. 'Do you really think you can help then?' he asked.

'Yes, I do, but only if you lose at least twenty kilograms in the next six months,' I said, turning back to Mrs van der Merwe. 'Otherwise, you are still going to have those operations.'

'How am I going to do that? I've been this weight for over thirty years and I hardly eat a thing now.' I saw a little smile flicker over her husband's face but he said nothing, wise man that he was. It's only people of small calibre who go on and on carping.

'A patient of mine lost fourteen kilograms in ten weeks on this new diet,' I said, writing on one of my letterheads in such a way that she could not see. I folded the paper and put it in an envelope, sealing it. 'Please don't open this before you get home. If you are serious about avoiding those two operations then follow my directions closely. Remember, total hip replacements are quite good, but knees are much more difficult. Your friend probably died from a fatty *embolus*. There is a lot of fat in the large bones of the leg and sometimes a clot may be carried in the blood to the heart, lungs or even the brain.' Dr van der Merwe nodded, approvingly.

'If you are determined to go through with it, then please phone and make an appointment for about a week's time because there are other important parts of the diet that we need to talk about.' I shook hands with them both and saw them to the door.

Mrs van der Merwe was back a week later. 'Very funny aren't you?' she said with a smile. '"Shut my mouth diet", indeed! Do you really think I can do it? I live to eat, you know!'

'There's nothing new in that, Mrs van der Merwe. I think it was Socrates who first coined the alternative: that one should eat to live, and not live to eat,' I replied.

She grimaced.

'Of course you can to do it. It will be tough, but I promise you, not nearly as tough as those two ops are going to be. Do it!'

'Okay, then,' she said, thinking about it, weighing up whether she really wanted to. She did want to, she told me later, but doubted that she had the willpower? 'What are the other parts of the diet?'

'I'm impressed. Many of my obese patients wouldn't do this, but I promise you, in six months' time, you will be a different person. You will have less pain, and you will be able to get out of chairs and in and out of cars much more easily. Stairs will cease to be the nightmare that probably now confronts you every day.' I looked at her questioningly.

She nodded, confirming what I had said. 'My husband has promised me a whole new wardrobe of clothes. That would be nice,' she finished, trying to convince herself.

'You can shop until you drop!' I said, trying to be funny. 'I promise you, you won't be sorry. Quite likely you will get off those blood pressure pills, too. The spin-offs from this diet will amaze you.

'Okay, so what must I do?'

'Firstly, go and buy a good quality juice extractor. Every day you must have at least one glass, preferably two, of fresh vegetable juice. Dilute it with water into two glasses. In it you must have at least two carrots and one celery stick and any other vegetables that are in season. Those large zucchini squash are excellent, cabbage is fine, and perhaps part of a leek or a spring onion. In fact, get busy in your garden. The more veggies you can grow yourself the better.'

She nodded making a few notes. 'Is it going to be quite expensive then?'

'Not at all. In fact, you will save money. Then one day a week, I want you on a complete juice or water fast. Freshly squeezed orange juice, apple juice, plums, or just the vegetable juice will be fine. The wider the spread of juices the better, or just a water fast if you like. Make it a quiet day at home as you may feel quite weak and trembly. You might be headachy, too.'

'Is that all?'

'No, then comes the difficult part. For three weeks in the month I want you on a very low protein diet. Low meat, low eggs and cheese, and you're not to splurge in the fourth week. The rest is fairly obvious and you know it yourself. Cut out fatty fried foods, sweet pastries, cakes and soft drinks. Look upon it as a new way of eating for the rest of your life. Heaps of fruit, salads and vegetables.

'Low protein!' she exclaimed. 'I thought high protein diets were the best way to lose weight.'

'They work but I don't think they are safe. It's harder this way, but healthier.'

'Twenty kilograms! How long will it take!

'You should try and do it in three to four months but if it takes you six, that's fine. Don't expect me to bully you; you have chosen to do this, so go and do it. Faith in yourself is usually the safest course in life.'

'I'm sorry, but I have no faith in myself!' She pulled a face.

'Think of it as a simple 'either/or', Mrs van der Merwe. *Either* lose the weight, *or* have the operations, with all the pain and potential complications. Phone me if you want advice and can I see you in four months' time, please,' I finished, trying to dismiss her. I had my doubts too that she would do it and, in any event, my next patient was waiting.

'Four months time! I thought you were going to treat my knees as well.'

'You are going to have to earn that treatment, Mrs van der Merwe. It will only be temporary relief, in any case, unless you lose the weight so, after you have lost the weight, we will start the treatment on your knees. Go on with those simple exercises, though.' I also gave her a list of supplements to take. 'Cod liver oil and that chondroitin sulphate, too, please.'

The next few months of Mrs van der Merwe's life were amongst the worst any person can ever experience, but it had nothing to do with her diet or her knees. Six months had passed, and I never heard from her, so I assumed that she went for the total knee replacements, but I was wrong. That she stuck to the 'shut your mouth diet' gamefully and lost the weight in under the four months was a credit to her, but Mrs van der Merwe had no inclination to go out shopping for those new outfits. When she finally arrived for a consultation, her clothes hung limply on her, and I could see without weighing her that she had lost all twenty kilograms. What I didn't understand was the sadness and loss of sparkle in her eyes. It made no sense. I expected her to be bursting with enthusiasm.

'Well done, Mrs van der Merwe, you are a star. Now, what's happening that's making you so glum?'

'My husband. He died three weeks ago.'

'Dead!' I couldn't believe it.

She nodded. 'Amyotropic Lateral Sclerosis,' she finished lamely.

I was stunned. 'I have never heard of the disease progressing that fast,' I exclaimed, thinking of his strange voice. The disease must have started in the nerves to the voice box. 'When was it diagnosed?'

'Three months ago.'

I didn't say anything for a few moments. What can one say? Eventually I simply said: 'I'm sorry. That is awful.' Not an accent, not polyps in the nose… but ALS, one of the most awful diseases to inflict mankind. *Lou Gerig's disease.** There is no known cause for the disease, nor is there any treatment. The motor neurons supplying the muscles of the body gradually disintegrate so the muscles atrophy and die. The brain, however, remains crystal clear, and the patient knows full well what is happening, particularly one who is a doctor. It is the epitome of an utterly humiliating disease, as victims can sometimes live for years, hopelessly crippled, unable to do even the most simple of tasks. Doctor van der Merwe chose otherwise. He joined his wife on the fast, only he didn't fast for one day a week. He followed it assiduously every day.

Mrs van der Merwe never had her operations. She consulted me a few times for treatment for her knees, and then cancelled. I wasn't sure whether to contact her, and in the end busyness drove her into the background of my mind. It was a full eighteen months later that the vertigo drove her back to the chiropractor. 'I'm dizzy again, Dr Preston. Can you adjust my neck, please?'

She had kept the weight off, and I was astonished how much her blood pressure had dropped but I was not surprised how much more easily she moved about. Wallenberg's test was still vaguely positive, and I went through the struggle again. Should I adjust her neck? I did, and she got over the dizziness very quickly, fortunately.

'I've brought you a small gift,' she said, when she arrived for her second consultation, package in hand.

'That's very kind of you. What is it?'

'You'll have to open it to find out?'

---

* Famous baseball player in the 1930s smitten by ALS. Remembered for his famous last words spoken to fans in the Yankee stadium: 'I consider myself the luckiest man on the face of the earth.'

I carefully opened the package. It felt like a picture frame. It was. A beautiful sketch of the leaning tower of Pisa. I was elated, thinking of the Pisa sign.* 'How did you know I was so interested in the tower of Pisa? Where on earth did you get this?'

'I sketched it, of course.'

'You did?' My mouth dropped open. 'I didn't know you were an artist. You must have done this years ago!'

'Look more carefully!'

In the bottom right corner were her initials, and the date. Two months ago. 'I'm sorry, but I don't understand. Did you do it from a photograph?'

'No, silly, I sat in the square and sketched it. Two months ago when I was on my trip around Italy.'

'You went to Italy! With those knees, at eighty!'

'After my husband died, I was very miserable for two months. To be honest I nearly took an overdose of pills several times. Then my daughter dragged me off to live with them which was about the worst thing that I could have done. They started treating me like a child, making me really fed up.'

'And then?'

'My son lives in England. He gave me a subscription for an artist's magazine called *The Artist* for Christmas, and I found an advert for a tour to Italy. So I joined them.'

'Your daughter, or your son, went with you?'

'No, of course not. I didn't want them bullying me, telling me I was far too old, and that I must rest up. That was the whole point, to escape from them!' she exclaimed.

'But, but... you mean you went on your own?'

'Yes, on my own. You're as bad as my children. Just because I'm old, and I've got bad knees, doesn't mean I'm an invalid! I had a wonderful tour, and I did this for you while we were in Pisa!' She was exasperated with me.

---

* Reference: *Frog in my Throat.*

Chapter Twenty-Three

JUST REWARD?

Men may not get all they pay for in this world,
but they certainly pay for all they get.

Frederick Douglass

Unlike many Black youths, Sipho Khoza had none of the inferiority complex that two generations of Apartheid had inflicted on many South Africans, black and white. His eyes were bright and he looked at me confidently, even insolently. *What do you have for me, White man?* He had little faith that this strange doctor's treatment could have a propitious effect on his health, but pain finally drove him in my direction; pain for which medicine had provided no satisfactory answers, though it had undoubtedly saved his life when he was a small boy.

Sipho's upper back had given him trouble for as long as he could remember: a deep aching pain that sometimes grew to an intolerable crescendo. At sixteen, he was a tall, thin lad, not malnourished, just slender in the Zulu tradition.

His English was good. That too was unusual. An inferior educational system had done its best to ensure that the Black youth remained inferior. *Carriers of water and hewers of wood* was the curse that Noah, the grand old man of the Bible, had placed on the descendents of his son Ham. It was no coincidence that Black education in South Africa was mostly awful, with only a few pockets of excellence: Apartheid ideologists had carefully crafted it that way, despite smooth assurances of 'separate but equal'.

It stemmed actually from the plain bad theology of religious zealots who were under the fanatical conviction that all doctrine could be neatly divided into two kinds: that which was their own and all other that should be neatly bundled together as Communistic, false and dangerous. They were the hands of God, carrying out the curse that He had placed on the descendants of Ham.

Ardent dogmatists would say it confirms the need for the study of doctrine: the curse on Ham wasn't of God, it was that of a drunken old fool, found naked by his son. Ham kindly covered his father with a blanket but, like all fathers, Noah had not appreciated being found out. Education for the races in South Africa was separate and very unequal, and largely remains that way, even ten-plus years post-Apartheid.

A Black boy predestined to a life of ignorance and pain. Bad medicine had certainly provided no answers. Actually that is probably unfair: good medicine had saved Sipho's life from the Tuberculosis bacillus when he was only two. The question, of course, was whether good medicine, and now Chiropractic had any better solutions for the debilitating pain that plagued him.

Sipho had one big leg up in life: a mother who drove herself mercilessly so that she and her son could escape from the ignorance that they were destined to. Deserted by a boyfriend once he discovered that she was pregnant with his child, Miriam Khosa had not been satisfied with the cards that life had dealt her. Having a grandmother in the true African tradition of *Ubuntu** did help: the old lady cared for baby Sipho while Miriam studied late into the night to become a teacher, whilst working in the day as a domestic help to keep body and soul together. The kindly white madam did help Miriam with her college fees.

---

* An ancient African word, meaning 'humanity to others'. Ubuntu also means 'I am what I am because of who we all are'.

After graduation it was some years before Ms Khosa was promoted to headmistress of a small Black community school where she drove her staff with the same flame that burnt in her own soul. After no more than a few short years, theirs was one of the very few schools to get a hundred per cent pass rate in the matriculation exam. Sipho had been privileged to learn excellent English from his mother who insisted on speaking to him only in the universal language of the world. It was she who taught him that faith in oneself is usually the best and safest course. Sipho had unlimited self belief.

Then tragedy struck. Mrs Khosa was murdered when Sipho was only ten, by a teacher she had fired: he flatly refused to make any attempt to meet the standards she demanded of her staff. Fortunately, knowing that life in South Africa is cheap, Mrs Khosa had the foresight to take out an adequate life insurance policy. Sipho had access to some of the things that White South Africans take for granted. It included Chiropractic care.

The positives of excellent health are additive. So are the negatives of a poor lifestyle: the smoker who is obese; the diabetic who won't exercise; the workaholic who won't take proper holidays. They rarely make old bones. Sipho also had many negatives in his young life and they added up to pain; bodily pain and mental anguish for him, but other sorts of pain for those around him.

'What's the trouble, Sipho?' I asked.

'I have pain in my neck and my back.'

'When did it start? Do you remember?'

'As long as I can remember.'

'Have you been to a doctor? Did they give a diagnosis?'

'Yes, I have been many times to the hospital. They said I have had tuberculosis. There is nothing they can do, I must just take painkillers.'

'Do you know when you had TB?'

'Yes, when I was a baby. I had an operation.' Sipho took off his shirt, and showed me an ugly scar in the mid back.

The poor child, I thought with a shudder. In most of the world TB is a well controlled, almost non-existent disease, but in South Africa, partly because of AIDS, it is rampant. Bone pain from spinal TB is excruciating, and he must have suffered terribly as a child.

'Sipho was very sick when he was about a year old. His mother took him to the hospital,' contributed his guardian.

I nodded. Excellent medicine had correctly diagnosed and treated the problem, releasing the abscess with an operation. That was all more than ten years ago, back in the Apartheid era when, ironically, basic medicine was available to the poor for no charge. The medical records that Sipho brought with him from the hospital concluded that there was no active TB.

As I went through the active and passive ranges of motion of his neck and upper back, and did the orthopedic and neurological tests that every chiropractor would use, two things were interesting: There was no spinal movement in two distinct areas of Sipho's spine; one where the tuberculosis bacilli had destroyed and fused the bones of his upper back, and another in the lower neck. The other interesting finding was that orthopedic testing proved that the pain he was experiencing came from neither area: it emanated from the area in between, at the level of the second and third thoracic vertebrae. I had no idea whether I could help him, but clearly new x-rays were indicated.

Fortunately for Sipho, the insurance policy that his wise mother had taken out to care for her son, in the event of her premature death, was more than adequate. Perhaps she had a premonition. Not many Black children could afford any form of treatment outside of the rudimentary hospital system, but Sipho's guardian indicated that there would be no problem. Sipho could go for x-rays and payment of my fees would not be a problem.

The x-rays were a shock. Not only was the area in the midback totally distorted by the tuberculous disease but, in the lower neck, Sipho had an unusual condition. Three vertebrae were fused together to form what are called 'block vertebrae'. It is a fairly rare congenital condition, nothing to do with the TB, but the chances that they occurred simultaneously in the same person were of the same order of magnitude as winning the jackpot. Two areas of Sipho's spine were fused solid as concrete, one by disease, and the other by a condition that he was born with. Orthopedic and Chiropractic testing indicated that the pain came from the area in between, where there were obviously excessive stresses on his young spine. Two significant negatives that added up to pain.

'I think I can help you, Sipho,' I explained to the young man, and his guardian. 'Just how much I am not sure. Perhaps fifty per cent, maybe more. There will be three phases of the treatment. In the first which will last about four to six weeks, I hope to be able to reduce your pain considerably. In the second, or rehabilitative phase, there will be less treatment from me, but many exercises to strengthen the area. I'm afraid I cannot cure this condition, no one can, so in the third phase you will have a treatment every six to eight weeks in attempt to control the situation. That is the best I have to offer. If it doesn't work out, then I promise to be honest with you, but you can expect it to be difficult. There will be no miracles; we will both have to work hard.'

'This TB has nothing to do with AIDS?' Sipho's guardian wanted to know.

'I doubt it,' I replied. 'He had the infection a long time ago and, if he was infected by the HI virus, then I would have expected to see other signs of AIDS by now.' Turning to Sipho I asked: 'You don't suffer from diarrhoea, or fungal infections?'

He shook his head.

'In all other respects you seem to be a fit, healthy young man, Sipho.' In theory, I was right but, in practice, quite wrong. 'Do you have any questions about the treatment plan?' They shook their heads.

The treatment went according to plan as I treated Sipho's spine over the following weeks. Another negative in Sipho's young spine was a 9 mm short right leg, giving him a significant scoliosis, aggravating his neck pain. That was easily dealt with. Fortunately he had the kind of scoliosis that could be remedied by a simple heel lift. Within six weeks Sipho declared that the pain in his back had indeed been reduced by about a half. He was satisfied and so was I, though there were a few surprises along the way.

'You've got some blood on your shirt, Sipho. What happened?'

'Oh, that's nothing. I had a little fight.'

'A fight?'

'We have a very cocky boy in our class. He is always asking for trouble, so I gave it to him.'

'Let me have a look.' The 'little fight' had given Sipho quite a nasty gash on the chest that was still oozing blood. I bathed it, careful to use gloves, thinking back to my childhood of the styptic stick that my father had used when shaving.

'How did this happen?'

'He pulled a knife on me. So, of course, I had to use my knife.'

I grimaced. 'Why on earth do you boys take knives to school? This is so dangerous, you could have been killed.'

Sipho grinned. 'He won't cheek me again. He's in hospital!'

The next month it was much the same. Sipho had a broken bone in his hand. 'What happened, Sipho?' I asked as I taped up his finger.

'Oh, it was just a stick fight after school. Nothing much.'

'But look at your hand. How can you say it is nothing?'

'You should see the other boy!'

'Don't tell me. I don't want to hear. How is your back doing?'

'It hasn't been so good this week. I have been getting headaches. Do you think it is coming from my back? I've been feeling quite tired lately.'

I examined him carefully. The part of his neck that might cause headaches was reasonable. He didn't have a temperature, and his blood pressure was fine. I gave him an adjustment, wondering if there was something else causing Sipho's headaches.

The weeks turned into months. Eventually Sipho was faced with his final matriculation exams. 'How has your back been with all the studying, Sipho? Are you still getting those bad headaches?'

Sipho gave me a broad grin. 'I'm tired of school, but it's nearly finished now.'

'And next year? What are your plans?'

'The White lady who teaches me Mathematics thinks I could go to the university. We look after her. Some of the *tsotsis*[*] have tried three times to steal her car, but we sorted them out.' He winked.

Sipho fiddled with his cap. I hadn't noticed it before, but he kept putting it on, and taking it off, and turning it one way or another. 'Your back? Those headaches?'

'My back is quite good, but I am very tired. I study late every night. I think that is the cause. The headaches have been bad this week.'

---

[*] Young thugs.

'I think you should go to the hospital. Get a check up. Your neck is really quite good.'

'The hospital! You think I am mad? More pills! I don't ever want to go there again.' He fiddled with his cap again. It was bright red.

'That's a new cap.' I could hardly have missed it.

'Yes, it's a fine cap, isn't it? I won it in a competition.'

'Congratulations, Sipho. That's very nice. Well done. Now that the exams are here, I should see you each week until they are over. There will be lots of extra stress. Then we can go back to a treatment every two months. Now remember the most important rule: *read the question carefully* in these exams. You can write many pages, but if you don't answer the question, then you will fail.' Sipho nodded.

I don't make much time for the newspaper. Five minutes for the headlines, even less for the sports page, and then a quick scan through the snippets. The first was from Switzerland: Orthopedic surgeons expected 25,000 broken legs that year during the ski season. Many surgeons work for five months, and then take off the rest of the year. I sighed. What a life. The second snippet had me shaking my head in disbelief: The boys in the matric class at Amakolwe High School had organized a new and unique competition: At the beginning of the year they had bought a bright red cap. The first boy to sleep with each girl in his class would win the cap. Class leaders declined to say who had won the trophy.

Chapter Twenty-Four

A RETREAT – AND AN ADVANCE

When one sits still and tries to focus, the mind becomes turbulent. It mounts its horse and starts galloping in all directions, north and south, into past and future, to places real and imaginary. Gradually, though, it does begin to be reined in. There are calmer moments too.

Anu Garg

You may be wondering how I escaped the attentions of the black dog after that epic visit to our summer holiday chalet at Lake Pastel. Two years passed before my election to chairman of the local Chiropractic branch, during which time I eventually came to myself, not without considerable prodding by the good wife, and others concerned at my downward slide; but first…

Of course, I know that depression and indecisiveness go hand in hand, where others are concerned that is, but I couldn't see my own blindness. There are naturally none so blind as those who will not see, so Helen started making some decisions on my behalf; like sending me on the retreat. The journey inwards proved long and arduous.

I had, in the past, been very cynical about retreats. What I needed in life was advances, not retreats, and the shallowness of my own spirituality did not allow for the many paradoxes that make up the life of faith. So, shortly after our disastrous return from Lake Pastel, Helen booked me in for a four-day silent retreat with our priest, using the Old Testament book of Micah as the focus. Something snapped that day when our neighbour recognized my face in the newspaper he was about to use to start the barbecue. All the good work started by the bat seemed to have been undone.

Four days of silence! Who on earth was Micah anyway. Only a Bible and a note book, and a hymn book, if Bernie wanted, were allowed. He didn't want. Not the hymn book, nor the retreat. For several days Bernie sulked and refused point blank to go: four whole days of going backwards in life. But, of course, 'she who must be obeyed' got her way in the end so, ten days after their Mount Pastel holiday, Bernie found himself driving to a hitherto unknown destination at the seaside.

The journey itself was a nightmare. Several times I nearly turned round and drove home but something drew me on and, in any event, the three other retreatants in my car were relying on me for the lift. I had reached rock bottom by then, so what was there to lose? The climb up the healing ladder had certainly begun at Lake Pastel but that final barbecue had turned it into a game of *Snakes and Ladders*.* Unable to sleep I was again back at *square one* and I knew it.

The retreat house came as a surprise. Set high on a cliff overlooking the ocean, it was not a house but one of those la-di-da mansions with seven en suite bedrooms, all with spectacular views overlooking the sea. A narrow set of steps cut into the virgin rock led down to a sandy beach that was open only for a few hours on either side of low tide. The regular thud-thud-thump as the waves crashed into the cliff face far below reminded us, if we woke in the night, where we were. I did not miss the irony that our place of retreat should be named *Voorwaarts.*† Forwards!

---

* Children's board game played with a dice. If you land on a snake you must go downwards, and a ladder takes you upwards.

† 'Forwards' (Afrikaans)

Standing on the wide veranda, the salt air fresh on my cheek and a hint of Frangipani in the air, I began once again to relax. I felt like a noviciate, a rank beginner in the matter of self-awareness, but the other retreatants I knew were rather more mature in the Faith. It was only years later that I was able to recognize the wisdom of Bertrand Russell, that it is only fools and fanatics who are so certain of themselves, the wiser being so full of doubts. This was no place for beginners. We sat at the round table on that first night, the conversation quiet and apprehensive, each knowing that, the moment they left the table, they were going into four whole days of total silence, broken only for one merciful hour each day with our priest, Bob. Images of monasticism leapt into my mind. 'Where is the bed of nails?' I asked. There was a twitter of nervous laughter. 'Fortunately no cold cloisters for us, but you could wear a robe of horse-hair,' a fellow retreatant smiled. None of us were in a rush to leave the table, secure in its fellowship, knowing that we would be totally alone once we left. There was an unusual camaraderie; most of us were tense.

Suffice it to say that which happened in Bernie's soul during the next four days cannot be readily recorded in a few brief pages. In the silence, dust of varying degrees of filth, that had been quietly swept under the carpet for decades and conveniently ignored, began to emerge in a disconcerting manner. In the prolonged silence Bernie could not avoid facing many issues that had long been sidelined. Undealt with issues, many of them long forgotten and deeply buried in his subconscious, were bogging Pilgrim's progress through life, weighing heavily on his mind and spirit. He was to discover that human growth sometimes, perhaps even regularly, requires silence and solitude, painful though these might be. This was not going to be an easy four days. Tears would be shed. Bernie was not normally a tearful man but advance in his life first demanded remorse. Although not immediately evident, but before the retreat was over, a new peace touched his life as he gradually came to terms with himself. It brought with it a new wisdom too, though it was only others that would perceive it. Bernie was painfully aware of his shortcomings and self-doubt hovered not far below the surface.

The first breakfast was a nervous hour as we all faced the beginning of what was obviously going to be an arduous affair. Not for the faint-hearted and even the normally unflappable Bob was looking strained. Spending an hour with each of seven neophytes, searching the bottoms of their murky ponds, rather like police divers looking for a dead body, giving each direction and comfort, was going to stretch him too. This was not going to be a picnic for any of us. Not a word was said, other than the grace we chorused together. Mostly, I found that my fellows were sensitive to my needs at table but once I had to get up and walk around to the far side of the table for the salt. It irritated me. At high school I would have kicked my neighbour on the shins but that did not seem appropriate at a retreat. What was I doing here? I was angry that Helen had cajoled me into it.

'Bernie, like the rest of Shafton, I know something of what has been happening in your life,' Bob said at our first short session. 'Helen has also been to see me, as you know, and she has filled me in with a few details. I also saw the tiny paragraph in the *East Griqualand Herald*, recording that the Board had found you not guilty of any misconduct with that schoolgirl. Today I would like you to read the whole of the book of Micah – it's only seven pages in your Bible – and then read these two verses several times over.' He passed me a slip of paper. 'Take your time with the passage, stay with it, and make notes of your progress. Okay? Any questions?' I had none. Half of me was irritated, that part which was used to giving the instructions and generally ordering people around, but the other half was slowly becoming more honest. Whilst I was a somebody in my professional world (or, at least I used to be), here I perceived myself as a nobody and I didn't resent being directed.

There was that word 'progress' again and Bernie couldn't help making a connection with Pilgrim. Pilgrim had a difficult day of it. A restless creature, he strode several times up and down the ninety-two steps to the beach, walking the sandy shore, passing other equally stressed individuals, giving only a curt nod of recognition. The reading of the seven chapters of Micah took less than an hour, and the re- 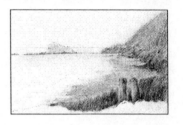 *reading of the two verses given by Bob, several times over, only a few minutes. What to do with the rest of the day?*

The rest of the day was characterised by denial. Hadn't the Board found him not guilty? Did his accountant not take responsibility for the grey areas of tax avoidance? The many hours spent soaring, away from family and patient responsibilities, weren't they his right? He indulged in a few minutes of day-dreaming, thinking of his friends soaring in their gliders high above the midlands on that glorious Saturday. Resolutely, and not without difficulty, he dragged his thoughts back to poor Pilgrim and his progress. The beautiful men and women whose bodies he touched on a daily basis, was that not his work? What was this about a pardoning God? He hadn't committed any serious transgressions. The odd thought, maybe.

'Bernie, how long have you been a Christian?' Pastor Bob asked me at our second session.

'Since I was nineteen. About thirty years,' I answered resentfully. I was *gatvol* with the retreat. 'Bob, I think I want to go home. I'm not cut out for this sort of thing.'

'Yes, it's a bit scary, isn't it? Did you ever sing that Negro spiritual: *Run to the rocks, rocks won't you hide me?* Stay with it, Bernie, you won't be sorry.' I couldn't see it then, but he was right. Later, I was not sorry.

'Oh, I don't know Bob. I'm finding this very boring.'

'Yes, that's where it always starts for everybody, Bernie, but there's worse to come, I'm afraid. If yesterday was boring as you were forced to get out of overdrive, then today will probably be disturbing.' He knew he had me. I couldn't turn and run and today was going to be a crunch day. 'Go back to verses 18 and 19 from yesterday for an hour or two. Then I want you to spend the rest of the day with these two verses from chapter 7.' He handed me another slip of paper. 'Make notes if there is any movement.' We prayed briefly together and I went off with my Bible and notebook. Page one, day one was blank.

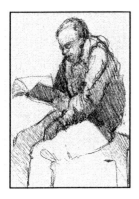

It was indeed a disturbing day for Bernie. God came walking through his creation looking for a ripe fig and a bottle of vintage red wine – and there was none to be found. Godly men had perished from the earth. Bernie spent the day wondering what it meant to be a godly man and what it was that God expected to find in Bernie's garden on that summer day? He spent the time alternately walking aimlessly on the beach, watching the rhythm of the waves, or carelessly sitting, Bible and notebook in hand, under one of the Giant Fig trees that proliferated along the coast. A pair of Knysna Louries kept him entertained for a while as they gorged themselves on the

tiny figs. Obviously the beautiful model was still fresh in Bernie's mind and, in general, his relationship with dozens of beautiful people came under the spotlight of that gaze that he was trying to escape.

My third session with Pastor Bob went a lot deeper. It is a disturbing fact that many doctors in general, and perhaps chiropractors in particular, because of our hands-on treatment, divorce the gentle does of their youth, who had supported them so faithfully through the tough years of training and the early stressful days of practice, only to go chasing after pretty nurses and patients. In their defence, sometimes it's the doctor who is the prey.

'Bob, when does a relationship become adulterous? What is adultery anyway?' I started off with what appeared superficially a rather facile question.

Bob looked at me, incredulously. 'Bernie, you have been a Christian for thirty years, married for nearly as long to the same woman, and you ask what is adultery?'

'Yes, that's what I'm asking,' I replied, angrily, frustrated.

He was non-plussed and didn't know where to start. So I helped him, continuing: 'Is it simply going to bed with another woman? Is it just a matter of sex?'

I suspected that he couldn't see what I was driving at, but Bob, being the patient and intuitive priest that he was, gave me the credit for a serious question: 'Go on, Bernie.' He wasn't being evasive but I could see from the way his dark brown eyebrows knotted together and the slight frown that creased his forehead that he was puzzled.

'Well, if I enter into a relationship with another woman – or man, for that matter – or several people, where there is a deep touching of minds and spirits, but it is strictly non-sexual, is that okay?'

Bob pondered my question for a few moments. 'Tell me about this touching of minds and spirits?'

'Let's say that a woman consults me with a condition that requires a course of treatment. Many spinal conditions are not going to be cured, and will require an initial course of treatment, often followed by years of maintenance and rehabilitation. During this time I become attracted to this woman's ideas, her intellect, her spirituality perhaps and, yes, maybe even her body. Let's just say that in some way or other she is a particularly beautiful person and we are attracted to each other. But, at this stage anyway, it's strictly platonic.'

'And then? What happens then?'

'Mostly nothing, but it's fertile ground.'

'And what is the physical part of this relationship?' Bob asked.

I thought for a moment: 'I would be touching some part of her. Mostly an area that hurts, part of her shoulder or neck, or the buttock or back. You know.'

'How would you describe this touch?' Bob persisted.

'It would be a healing touch. Sometimes it may be painful, often light and sensitive. Sometimes we would be very close, physically I mean, but mostly with her back to me. Occasionally it might be with an intimate part of her body, as in reducing a subluxated coccyx, which sometimes has to be done rectally, but then I always ask my secretary to come into the room, or reducing a rib which might have to be done through the breast tissue. Obviously the lingering touch is verboten but sometimes, Bob, occasionally this relationship is like intercourse, but with nothing but a layer of aromatic oils between us, and a flow of thoughts and ideas. Orgasmic in a non-sexual way, if you know what I mean.'

Bob frowned. He didn't like the simile.

'In all this, what is your relationship with Helen like?'

'Mm, mostly pretty good. She is a good woman, a fine mother, and a wonderful cook. I love her but we know each other pretty well now, and I suppose meeting a new mind is stimulating. Perhaps we know each other too well and are a bit bored with each other but we are comfortable together and there is no embarrassment when we are alone.'

'Do you still sleep together?'

'Yes, we do but we're not likely to empty the *acorn jar*!'[*]

'So what's really your question, Bernie?' He didn't ask about the acorn jar.

I thought about that for a while. 'Well, I've been struggling with this meeting of minds. I don't sleep with my patients obviously but I find their ideas and thoughts very stimulating. I enjoy their company, perhaps even more than Helen's sometimes. I worry about it. You know Bob, I feel I really get to know them? Deeply, intimately. There's no conquering, no violation, no possessing, but I feel that I really *know* them. When it says in the Bible, Bob, that Abraham *knew* Sarah, does it just mean that they just slept together? Is it just something carnal? Or did he really know her? Is knowing just about sex? I almost feel that I have committed adultery with some of these patients, yet I've never even touched them indecently. Is that crazy, Bob? What does it mean to be a godly man? I'm afraid of myself, Bob.' The anxious questions came thick and fast.

'To answer all those questions, Bernie, I want you to spend today with chapter 6, verse 8.' He passed me another of his little slips of paper.

I left my third session with Bob angry. I felt he had just dismissed me but, looking at my watch, I realized that the hour had sped by. My time was up. Why didn't he just give me a straight answer? It was only some months later that this new life coursing through my veins enabled me to see that,

[*] A fable in which it is suggested that if a couple put an acorn into a jar whenever they make love in the first year of their relationship, and take an acorn out thereafter, they will never empty the jar.

just as I had given no simple question, there was no straight forward answer. Wise man Bob wanted me to work out my own answers. With fear and trembling.

Justice and kindness and walking with God. Bernie walked angrily up and down the steps and was nearly caught by the incoming tide on the beach in his distraction. Gradually the thoughts crowding through his mind settled in a new cohesion: the only wrong-doing in his relationship with his patients was that gradually, simultaneously, as some of these intercourses with beautiful patients developed a new richness, his knowing of his own wife was fading. Was she being excluded? Were they becoming bored with each other? Had they fully explored their own partnership? Were they still growing? Together, apart, not at all? The matter of two women with whom Bernie had become just a little too intimate also came butting into his thoughts, disconcertingly, uninvited. One had slapped him, the other had started insisting on the last appointment of the day, until Bernie's prim and proper secretary cottoned on.

We shall here leave Bernie's 'progress' over the next two days. Suffice it to say, there were tears of remorse shed and a new weighing of the intersection of his private and public life. The passage given by Bob for the fourth day directed him towards a new 'looking to', and 'waiting for', to be added to the previous 'walking with' God. It was here Bernie realized that Bob was directing him for the answers he was seeking. He also revisited the passage from the first day and the 'casting of our sins into the depths of the sea' took on a new meaning.

One other seminal event occurred that should be mentioned. Whilst Bernie was floundering in a sea of despair one of the other retreatants began quietly singing that great hymn of the Faith, 'Amazing Grace'. Bernie knew about John

257

Newton. Captain of a slaving ship for some twenty years, Newton penned the words one stormy night at sea. Newton became one of the great champions of the Faith, and the anti-slavery movement. The hymn could not have come at a better moment for Bernie.

Retreat, or no retreat, the late evening cup of Milo was violently disturbed. There was a screeching of brakes and a very loud crash on the street outside the mansion. We hastily donned our day-clothes again and headed for the gate. It was not a pretty sight: a large, strongly built, old tank of a car had smashed at high speed into the back of a tiny papier-mâché car that had stopped at the traffic light outside the mansion. The little car and its occupants had been violently shoved thirty metres down the road into a brick wall.

I rushed back to my room for my emergency bag, shouting over my shoulder for Bob to get a wheel spanner or a heavy wrench. I saw one of the others rushing to the phone.

Bob and I raced down the street together with others close behind. The door of the car was locked and we couldn't open it. Peering through the windows we could see a young couple, obviously badly injured and unconscious.

'Petrol, Bernie. Can you smell the petrol?' shouted Bob.

'Use the wheel spanner, Bob. Smash the window!'

Using first a quite timid tap and then a mighty crashing blow Bob targeted the side-window which shattered, and I was able to put my hand through and unlock the door. Using the wheel spanner, and all our combined force between us, we managed to pry the door open. I heard a cry from one of the women behind me. It wasn't a pretty sight. The young man's head was badly crumpled and it was with great difficulty that we managed to drag him from the car, desperately disentangling his feet from the pedals. His right leg was obviously broken just above the ankle.

Bob by this stage had gone around to the passenger door, which I had managed to unlock from the inside.

'Careful, Bernie. The airbags could spring at any moment.' I hadn't thought of that. They were obviously faulty.

The girl had a safety belt on, which saved her life, and I managed to release it through the driver's door, but I could see her head and neck were at a strange angle. I could hear sirens wailing in the distance.

'Careful with her head, Bob,' I shouted, racing around to the other side. We were faced with a terrible dilemma. The smell of petrol was getting stronger all the time and I knew we could have a conflagration at any moment, but we had to be very careful with the girl. Gently cradling her neck and shoulders on my chest, one of the women stabilizing her head under my direction, we managed to drag her from the wreck just in time. As we laid her across the street on the pavement, the car exploded with a 'whump' and a flash of heat rocked us all back.

'What about the driver of the other car?' I shouted.

'I'm okay,' said a voice from behind me. I turned and saw a young man with a nasty gash on his forehead that was bleeding profusely, but otherwise he looked all right. I could smell the alcohol on his breath and had difficulty not reaching for the wheel spanner.

The paramedics arrived with their flashing lights and stretchers. I was glad to step back and let them take over. Within minutes they had gone with a roar of engines, their drips in place, sirens shrieking. We slowly made our way back to the retreat house. Two of the women, realizing they couldn't help, were on their knees. Several others were sobbing. Those directly involved were too shocked to say anything. I saw my hands and clothes were covered with the young man's blood and I took myself off to the shower. *Fool,*[*] I thought, *you didn't even take time to put on your*

---

[*] Over thirteen per cent of the HIV seropositive people in the world live in South Africa.

259

surgical gloves, Bernie. I carefully washed myself again and again, washing out not only the dirt and blood but trying to erase the images seared onto my brain. I wept for them, the tears coursing down my face along with the hot water, knowing that the news was not going to be good. It wasn't.

The final breakfast was a silent affair. Encouraged to talk normally again, prior to re-entering the real world, we were all lost in our thoughts. A call to the hospital had confirmed our fears: the young man was dead on arrival and the girl had a ruptured spinal cord. She would never walk again. Who was the most unlucky of the two? I was grateful that Bob didn't go through the 'God has given, God has taken away' routine. A drunk had violently snatched their lives away, not God, but He had allowed it. The only alternative is a world of robots unable to make choices, to please or disobey Him, a humanity void of the precious capacity of free will.

Bob invited each of us to each spend a weekly hour with him for the next month, to bring the retreat to completion. 'Bernie, I realize that human sexuality is something you are faced with on a daily basis, but was there something more behind your questions. I had the feeling you hadn't told me everything. Was it simply that girl and your other patients, or was there something else?'

I gulped. Was I so transparent or had he been given special insight? I wondered whether to talk about it. Would it set me free from my anger and fear?

'I once had a friend – he's dead now, killed I think, by what happened – whose wife developed the kind of relationship with our minister that I have with some of my patients. They were both wonderful people, intelligent, full of ideas and very spiritual. I knew them both well. My friend was in some ways a bit of a plod. None of us in the church would accept what was happening in front of our eyes, blind fools that we were, and gradually my friend and the minister's wife were excluded from this exciting new relationship. They were so spiritual, praying together and counselling those in difficulty. There couldn't be anything wrong with it, surely? Well, the inevitable happened.'

'What happened?'

'They all got divorced and the minister married my friend's wife.'

Bob wasn't so unshockable after all.

'When did the adultery actually happen, Bob? When did it begin? Assuming they only slept together after they were married, was it an adulterous relationship from the beginning? I'm afraid, Bob.'

'You already know the answer, Bernie. I don't have to tell you.' He stopped, thinking. I too was pondering his words. He was throwing all the responsibility back onto me, making me work.

'I have two questions for you this week, Bernie. First, is there a place in your heart, as there is in the heart of God, for the people who are not so beautiful? For the plods, and the drunks, and the adulterous ministers, and that girl who is going to be a paraplegic? What about them?'

I cocked my head, thinking, desperately trying to escape.

'Secondly, what are you going to do to enrich and re-inflame your marriage with Helen? That's the only way to conquer your fear of the beautiful people you have to touch on a daily basis.'

I left humbled by the wisdom of the man, thinking that, whilst Helen and I still went to the theatre, sometimes watched television together, read books and listened to music, we almost never spoke meaningfully to each other.

A wise retreat can sometimes be the start of a great advance.

Chapter Twenty-Five

A NEW CANVAS

*The greater danger for most people
is not setting our aim too high and falling short;
but in setting our aim too low, and achieving our mark.*

Michaelangelo

Boredom. The official number one complaint of teenagers in the developed world apparently, and not only teenagers. My usual thought is: *Take the profound step of selling your television and dump that DVD player in the Thames or the Tugela.* It may just create the space for something exciting to happen. Certainly one of the secrets of my profoundly interesting life has been to severely limit TV time.

I approached the passport control where a young woman took my passport and ticket, perused them, and gave them back to me without so much as a look at me. I saw the blank look in her eyes and wondered for a moment about the meaning of her life. Here were two human beings, in very close proximity and yet utterly unconnected. As I took the passport our fingers touched briefly but the connection was even less intimate than holding hands with a robot.

I watched her out of the corner of my eye for the next ten minutes; the utter inanity of her work life moved me. How can we do such things to human beings? No different I suppose to what happens in many factories: sew this zip onto those garments, fit this oil filter to that car or glue those soles onto these shoes.

I moved on to the baggage check-in desk. The reaction was different yet similar. The clerk preserved her sanity by chatting constantly to her neighbour in the next booth, and our connection was equally distant. Not once did our eyes meet as she looked at my passport and ticket, and checked in my baggage, not even checking that it was indeed my photo. The accumulation of my life had been condensed and was squeezed into a twenty kilogram suitcase, a laptop over my shoulder and a briefcase full of the documents needed to get me into Holland. That was all I needed. It was only some weeks later that I discovered that I wasn't going to Holland at all, but a province of the Netherlands where the proud people consider themselves anything but Hollanders.

At the security check point I found a young man who had perfected the art of preserving his sanity: he used humour. In front of me stood a young couple, she carrying their small child, perhaps four months old. Methodically they took off their jackets, their pouches and bangles, placing all in the baskets that go through the x-ray scanner.

'And the baby, too,' commanded the security official with a deadpan official-sounding voice. The couple looked uncertainly at each other, the young woman clutching her child more closely, whilst Dad reached for the child to put him in the basket. There was a twitter behind me in the queue and I, too, was appalled by the command. Just a few minutes earlier we had all heard him dealing mercilessly with a man who had tried to sneak a flick-knife onto the aircraft. The couple was dumbstruck. Unexpectedly, a broad smile crossed his face, and his loud guffaws had the whole departure hall looking our way. He reached over and touched the child's cheek, complimented the mother on her beautiful baby and ushered them on their way with not so much as a glance at their goods and chattels.

The move to the land of Windmills and Canvases was a sudden one, unexpected in that neither Helen nor I had thought of Europe, nor had we anticipated the frightening speed at which events would move. Four months and one week after receiving the letter of invitation to join a busy practice in Zuid Limburg that I found myself sitting on an airplane, terrified that we were making a dreadful mistake. Both my mother's family, and Helen's had been in South Africa for more than 150 years ago. Would I allow fear to shrink my life or could I let courage expand our horizons? 'We're only going for a few years,' we told everyone. 'The contract is only for three years.'

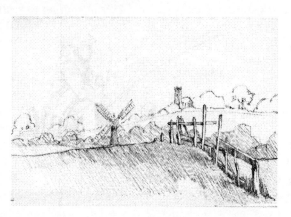

Yet the move was also expected. For some years Helen and I had watched with envy the way young adults leave and travel the world, and we had developed a sense of *we're going to do something like that*! Why should only the young be privileged to see the world? Were we too old? Over the hill? The first of two final straws, as yet unweighed at the time the invitation arrived, was our son's sudden departure to join a million South Africans living in London. The second was an unsolicited email that arrived on my computer: *The ratio of glider pilots in the Dutch population (1 per 1871) was the highest in the whole world.*

I had never been to Europe, Asia or Australia and I had visited only about ten American states. A deepening sense of being in something of a rut oppressed me. My world was not expanding, with more and varied experiences, nor getting smaller as many say, with distant parts reachable within a matter of hours. I had a sense that it was slowly shrinking, and I with it. A number of patients in those last few weeks in practice were angry. Who was going to look after them? There was talk of rats abandoning ship, and other comments by a people who felt they were being deserted by yet another emigrating doctor. I recalled the same feelings when our only orthopaedist Jeremy Thomas left Shafton for Australia: *should we too be going?* But one elderly farmer looked at me kindly and said: 'The only difference between a rut and a grave is the depth. If you must, Dr Preston, then go but please come back.'

'Of course, we are coming back, Mr van Tonder, it's only for three years.'

Bradley's comments were more disturbing: 'You won't come back, you know.'

'Nonsense, Bradley, of course we are coming back. I am only going on a three-year contract.'

'Mark my words: you won't be back.' Disturbing words. I hadn't even considered that possibility but, on reflection, I realized he could be right. I had worked hard at handing my patients over to colleagues, knowing that the continuing care was important, but Bradley's problems were so unique that I really didn't know how to pass him on. Treatment of Bradley's condition was so instinct-based and the feel of my hands that it was impossible to hand him over with any confidence.

'When did I first consult you?' Bradley asked.

I looked at my records: '1975. That was my first year in practice, young and naïve,' I said with a grin.

And naïve I was. It was only later that I recalled the sage words of advice given me by an elderly medical doctor: *'You probably won't miss important things in a new patient, but be very careful of the returning patient.'* Bradley had first arrived with a very sore low back which, in fact, turned out to be quite routine, but I made the mistake of taking only a shallow history of a serious neck injury that occurred some twenty years earlier.

'Remember the time I came back about six months later, and made your secretary and about five patients very angry?' Bradley laughed. Even though it was more than twenty years ago, I still clearly remembered the events of that day. Bradley arrived with a new condition, about which he hadn't warned Sally when he made the appointment. She had set aside only fifteen minutes for a routine consultation and I ended up running nearly an hour late.

When I walked through to my reception area, Bradley was sitting with head between his hands and his elbows on his knees. I was concerned. 'Come through, Bradley,' I said, wanting to shake his hand. He gave me a bleary look and I could see he was drugged to the hilt.

'I have a terrible headache, Doc. I've had it every day for a month and I just can't stand it any longer. Please, can you help me?'

I went through the usual questions: when did it start, was he in good health, were there any other sinister signs, had he seen his doctor, how many analgesics was he taking in a week, had he had any injuries? About an hour later I had finished and established that Bradley had been having these three-month headaches, every year or so, since a very serious car *trauma** in which he had fractured a bone in his neck, the *atlas*. That alone was enough to kill most people but Bradley was a survivor, carefully and thoroughly managed by an excellent neurosurgeon. He lay for six weeks in traction, followed by three months in a collar. The bone healed very adequately but the soft tissue damage and the traction on the

---

* Car trauma sounds quite awkward, but we should not avoid the fact that most MVAs are no accident; they are highly predictable.

nerve roots and the meninges* of the spinal cord continued to give him crippling headaches.

'How many painkillers are you taking, Bradley?' I asked.

'Five to ten a day,' he mumbled. I start to get excited when patients are taking more that about ten a week, and very excited when they are taking over twenty. In a recent screening of the Kidney Olympics (yes, I do watch TV sometimes), the dangers of over-medication had been burned onto my brain forever whilst watching young athletes who mostly had lost their kidneys through abuse of over-the-counter medication. Bradley was taking cocktails of over forty pills per week.

Complicating the problem was the fact that Bradley's blood pressure was significantly though not dangerously raised. No x-rays of his neck had been taken since the accident, and another surgeon had earnestly told him *never* to consult a chiropractor for his neck. It was far too dangerous.

X-rays and a CT scan confirmed what my hands had already told me. There were severe degenerative changes in the joint between the *atlas*, the first bone in the neck, and the *axis*, the second bone. The movement in the joint was reduced by over fifty per cent and the inflammatory changes were affecting the dura and the Greater Occipital nerve that supplies large parts of the scalp.

'Doc, these headaches usually stay for about three months, said Bradley. 'Nothing works. I should know: I've been having them for over twenty years.'

Bradley was truly suicidal. Could I help him? Would I help him? Did he have the right to Chiropractic care? Which was more important: his health or my reputation? Was I prepared to risk all, defying a neurosurgeon? All these questions came tearing at my conscience, overwhelming me.

---

* Membranes that cover the brain and spinal cord.

When treatment threatens to be more dangerous than the disease itself, I have always strongly believed the patient and family should be fully informed. They should weigh the facts, just as I had to. Were they comfortable with me adjusting Bradley's neck? Had *they* too heard the still, small voice confirming and giving me the green light to go ahead?

I started with a conservative and gentle programme of mobilization of Bradley's neck, soft tissue therapy, traction, various electrical gadgets and acupuncture and, of course, a consultation with his doctor concerning his blood pressure. Bradley was quite significantly overweight, gift of a job that kept him chained to a computer. His blood pressure stabilized nicely but there was absolutely no improvement in the headaches. In fact they got worse with my conservative therapeutic ministrations.

Finally the day came: 'Bradley, I am going to adjust your neck. As gently as I can. Are you both absolutely comfortable with that?' Bradley was not in a state to drive, so his wife Cynthia was taking a few hours off work to bring him. I looked at them both. They both nodded their heads. There was however another problem: there is sometimes no such thing as a gentle manipulation of a very degenerate joint. Gentle thrusts achieved absolutely nothing and finally I gave his neck a very solid adjustment. The resounding crack could have been heard on the street outside my window, and had them quite shocked. I wasn't afraid, just anxious.

It took only one adjustment. Bradley came in smiling the next day, the headache completely lifted. It could have ended differently. I decided against adjusting his neck again, and in fact it was not necessary for nearly another year. Chiropractors will argue long into the night as to whether such a neck should be regularly adjusted, but I decided to let sleeping dogs lie. Bradley knew the dangers of the adjustment of his atlas, which only rarely becomes an arthritic joint, and had tried all the supposedly safer treatments. Just how safe the 45 analgesics per week, in part prescribed for him, but supplemented by readily available over-the-counter medication is, of course, a moot point. All to no avail, in any case. His neck, nine months later when the headaches started again, was just as difficult to adjust, and I had to try various subtly different positions of the head to get a release. Again, once it gave a thunderous crack at the second consultation, his headache lifted within a few hours for yet another year. I didn't rush in, very conscious that I was walking where angels fear to tread.

How to hand over patients like Bradley to a colleague? The sense of guilt, of deserting people who relied on me, were amongst the first few tentative strokes on the new canvas that represented our new life in the Netherlands. Bradley's threat that I would not come back was etched in heavy black acrylic in one corner.

My first flight over central Europe was stunning. Although already past mid-summer the northern slopes of the Alps were still snow-covered. It was a remarkable dawn with a full moon setting in the west while the sun was making its presence felt in the east with a shepherd's warning. The contrasting red and grey sky was streaked with the vapour trails of dozens of large aircraft and the approach to Zurich was as beautiful as any I had ever experienced, even if I wasn't sitting behind the controls.

Moving to Holland for three years is probably the most stressful things I have ever done, until the language exam was passed, at any rate. 'Don't worry,' several people said, 'It will be just like Afrikaans,' the language that the descendants of the seventeenth century Dutch colonists still speak in South Africa. Nobody warned me until I arrived at the language school that Dutch is reputed to be the third most difficult language in the world. I got off the plane at Schiphol airport and eventually found my way into a small diner with several other tourists. I groaned when a large woman who had been particularly irritating on the flight sat down at my table, speaking loudly in Afrikaans. When the *ober* came to take the menu she ordered a second breakfast in the same loud irritating voice. I watched the look of dismay on the waiter's face with interest. Finally he said to her in accented but very understandable English: 'I'm afraid I don't understand a word you said, madam. Do you speak English?' Her family roared with laughter but she retorted in English: 'I am not amused,' probably unaware she was quoting a famous English monarch.

Had I known that my second patient was to be a small boy who had fallen down seven stairs in the night – Dutch staircases are nearly as dangerous as underpoliced South African roads – fracturing his skull and giving himself a *hersenschudding* (concussion) – I would probably have never come. Ah, these long Dutch words which were to tease me, but that is a story for my next book: *Goat in my Oesophagus*. The cheeses of the Netherlands, and especially that from their goats, and the yarns of their goat-keepers would be more than enough to fill another book, or cover a broad canvas, as my publisher calls it. The land of van Goghs and Esschers, of architects and water engineers, and the delightful Limburgers gave me plenty of scope to develop my own artwork. Surprising, I did not have one flight in a glider during those three years. I've already got that t-shirt.

Tot straks. [*]

---

[*] See you soon.

Afterword

FRIENDLY FIRE

(from *Goat in my Oesophagus*)

The most civilized people are as near to barbarism
as the most polished steel is to rust.
Nations, like metals, have only a superficial brilliancy.

Antoine de Rivarol

Anybody who has read any of my books will know that I am supremely interested in gaits – the way people walk. Not that there is anything new in that, but it fascinates me, and I have made a half promise to myself to make a video one day of the 101 ways in which patients walk. In fact I am so crazy about it, that I watch people in the shopping malls and supermarkets, and even occasionally ask a person in the street: 'Would you mind awfully if I asked you why you walk in that way?' Mostly I get replies like: 'I ran a marathon yesterday, and I have a blister on my heel'; or, 'Bugger off, can't you see I'm blind drunk!' Well yes, that may seem obvious, but ask any person with Multiple Sclerosis how many times they have been accused of being drunk, and you would be shocked.

There was no mistaking de heer van Onzelen's gait. Even the friend I have made on the bus recognized it. We were going home one evening – his name is Hendrik, he is the male equivalent of a Dutch char. He *poetsen's* – cleans houses. We watched Mr Onzelen struggle onto the bus. I nudged Hendrik: 'Why do you think he walks like that?' I whispered, while the object of our gaze was, out of earshot, flashing an *abonnement* (monthly bus card) at the driver.

'He's only got one leg, of course,' said Hendrik. I had to keep reminding him to stick to the queen's Dutch but, being a fairly simple fellow, with not much education, Hendrik kept slipping back into *dialect* or what the hoi-polloi call plat-Dutch. Each village in Limburg has its own dialect, more than 200 in all, most of them quite similar, some fairly similar to Dutch, but Hendrik might just as well be speaking Polish, for all my unaccustomed ear knew.

It's a tribute I suppose to what must be one of the most stable parts of the world, where old men plant trees, knowing they will never sit in their shade or eat of their fruit, but also knowing that, while the occasional apple may fall and roll away from the tree, most of the fruit falls and lies under their branches. They knew their children and their children's children would continue to enjoy the fruit of the cherry and apple orchards that they had been planting for hundreds and perhaps thousands of years in Limburg. I had to be careful: *appelvlaai en slagroom* (apple pie and whipped cream) was beginning to have an effect on my waistline. So local dialects spring up amongst a stable people, each village with its own accent, words and expressions. How the Dutch love their *uitdrukkings*. Sayings like: *Tall trees attract strong winds* and *I am standing with two feet in one sock.* I thought for a moment of men like Vincent van Gogh and Wim Duizenberg (president of the European Central Bank who was given the onerous task of convincing countries like France that they had to give up their devotion to the Franc in favour of the Euro) – very tall men who attracted a lot of flak, but remain giants of the Dutch landscape.

It wasn't too many weeks before I was last onto our bus, and only one seat remained: next to heer van Onzelen. *'Hoi-a,'* I greeted him, in the local plat. He gave me a suspicious look, typical of how the Dutch treat strangers, and replied: *'Hoi,'* and looked away. It only took one word out of my mouth and he knew that a crab-apple had rolled into Limburg. Of course, my silly woolly mohair cap knitted many years previously by a favourite patient also made it plain to everyone on the bus that this was no Limburger. (But it protects my ears from the strong Russian winds that sweep in from the east. Not that I have any ambition to be a tall tree.) I wasn't so easily put off, especially as I knew well by now that, once you get under the thick skin of the local people, they must be amongst the warmest-hearted people in the whole world.

'Do you work in Heerlen?' I asked in my poor Dutch, but having planned out the sentence carefully, I managed to get the form of the verb correct. 'I see you on the bus everyday.'

He looked up and I could see he was trying to evaluate this stranger. *Could I crack his shell?* Mostly I find that, once they know you are making a serious attempt to learn their language, they will open a small crack and let you in. 'Yes, I am a teacher in Heerlen,' came the guarded reply.

'I come from Zuidafrika so please excuse my bad Dutch,' I replied. That awoke some interest in him.

'Oh, and how long have you been here?' he asked.

'Nearly three months.'

'Then your Dutch is quite good,' he said. 'I suppose the Dutch dialect they speak in your land has helped.'

'I suppose it did help, though my Afrikaans* is actually very weak. I am an English-speaking South African.'

'Ah, a *rooi-nek*†,' he said with the first glimmer of a smile.

'Yes,' I grinned. 'You must have read some South African books.'

---

* Language still spoken in South Africa by the descendants of the Dutch.
† Red-neck. Mocking nickname for the descendants of the fair skinned English who still do not tolerate the African sun very well.

'But of course,' he said. 'I teach literature, and I love many of your writers. Some crazy ones too,' he finished darkly.

'Like who?'

'I have read some of Hendrik Verwoerd's writing, a genius of course, but like Carl Marx led the world – your world – down a very dark cul-de-sac.' I nodded, having to agree. 'But Deneys Reitz and Jan Smuts and your new Coetzee are the most wonderful writers.'

I was pleased to have read English translations of all three, but discussions in Dutch, outside of my very limited vocabulary was quite impossible. Religion, politics and literature were simply no-go areas. What I was really interested in was his gait!

'You've read *Disgrace*[*] then?'

'Yes, they tell me rape is a big topic in Zuidafrica.'

'I'm afraid it is.'

'No wonder you have such a problem with HIV!' I nodded. 'What brings you to Limburg?'

'I am a chiropractor. There's a big shortage here in the Netherlands.'

'Ah, a *kraker*[†],' he said with a broad grin. Finally I had got through the thick skin. I nodded again.

It wasn't for some weeks before I sat next to Mr van Onzelen again. He eyed me: 'Can you do anything for sore backs?'

'Sore back are my business. I deal with them all day long.'

'Have you got a business card?' he asked. I reached into my wallet. 'I lost my leg when I was nine years old,' he continued, looking out of the window. 'Landmine.'

---

[*] Disgrace by J.M. Coetzee won the Nobel prize for literature in 2003.

[†] Bone cruncher.

Chiropractic – Quo Vadis?

It is now over thirty years since I graduated from Chiropractic College and my journey as a health-care professional since then has probably closely mirrored that of Bernard Preston.

In that time there have been many significant changes to the profession that have been of benefit to the profession itself – but, more importantly, have been of particular benefit to our patients and the general public.

The introduction of low-force treatment techniques has meant that chiropractors now have a greater ability to deal effectively, safely and gently with the full range of patients – from tiny babies to the osteoporotic elderly – many of them in considerable pain – without fear of causing unnecessary further pain or harm.

The early 1970s saw the formation of an accrediting agency for Chiropractic educational institutions. Today, that body has international affiliates which all combine with common goals and standards to ensure that – no matter where a patient might be in the world – he or she can be confident that, when attending a chiropractor, that practitioner will have had a very similar standard of education to that of any other chiropractor – and equivalent to our colleagues in the medical professions.

The founding of a truly international body, the *World Federation of Chiropractic*, in 1988 has seen some 85 countries join together in dialogue and decision-making for the mutual benefit of chiropractors and their patients. A development of the concept underlying the formation of the European Chiropractors' Union in 1932, it seeks on a global scale to ensure that any legislation passed is similar to that in other countries, and that educational institutions in the process of providing Chiropractic education comply with the minimum educational requirement within a university-based curriculum. Now we have further strengthened our goals in this important area with the recent release of guidelines on Chiropractic education from the *World Health Organization.*

When I first graduated there was one (just one!) research study into the effectiveness of Chiropractic. Today, our profession has the most widely researched treatment for low back pain. New studies are continually being conducted into both the effectiveness and cost-effectiveness of our profession. The corollary is the improved treatment protocols for patients presenting today to chiropractors with a wide array of problems. I see this activity increasingly being the norm; and, as a result, Chiropractic continuing to be the treatment of choice by the general public for many common conditions.

The embracing of *evidence-based medicine* by chiropractors will inevitably lead to further steps being taken which will benefit patients. There will be further cooperative efforts between orthodox healthcare practitioners and chiropractors, leading to a 'team effort' to deal with common complaints. This is already apparent in the field of sports medicine where Chiropractic is being increasingly included in the world of football, rugby and the Olympics – to name but a few areas of involvement. This has been largely made possible by the formation of a specialist Chiropractic organisation called *Fédération Internationale de Chiropratique du Sport* – generally known as FICS. The efforts of this organisation to place Chiropractic within international sport have been wonderfully supported by numerous athletes from many disciplines who have personally seen the advantages of having chiropractors as part of their healthcare teams.

These are exciting times for the profession and it gives all of us involved in Chiropractic a great feeling to be able to play a small part in the advancement of the profession.

Dr Barry Lewis D.C. CCSP FCC(UK)
President
British Chiropractic Association